PATHOLOGICAL

The True Story
of Six
Misdiagnoses

PATHOLOGICAL

The True Story
of Six
Misdiagnoses

SARAH FAY

HarperOne
An Imprint of HarperCollinsPublishers

HarperCollins books may be purchased for educational, business, or sales promotional use. For information, please email the Special Markets Department at SPsales@harpercollins.com.

FIRST EDITION

Designed by THE COSMIC LION

Illustrated decorative designs and icons © Jamey Ekins/Shutterstock

Library of Congress Cataloging-in-Publication Data has been applied for.

ISBN 978-0-06-306868-1

22 23 24 25 26 FRI 10 9 8 7 6 5 4 3 2 1

For everyone who's been diagnosed—
and misdiagnosed and overdiagnosed

Contents

Prologue

The slower we walked, the more I seemed to sweat. Summer. Chicago. The two of us wandering the streets around Northwestern Memorial Hospital looking for the inpatient psychiatry unit where Dr. H said I could find help. I'd left him a message. He hadn't called back.

The buildings seemed dislocated and distant. Doctors and nurses in scrubs passed us on the sidewalk. Their voices cracked against my chest. A cab honked. A truck started up, billowing exhaust.

I heard the strain in your voice when you asked why the psychiatric unit wasn't where Dr. H said it would be. Worry weighed down the skin of your barely aging face. (People said you looked fifty though you were in your seventies.)

The families, people say. *The families go through hell.*

I'll never know what it was like for all of you. So much of that time I spent alone, trying to understand the six diagnoses I thought were real.

———

This isn't a classic mental-illness memoir. That kind of memoir is a quest story. From the beginning, our hero is exceptional. She's a debutante or a celebrity or a genius or at the very least she attends an Ivy League school when her enviable potential is dashed by mental illness. Her journey is extreme. She must leave the ordinary world in search of the elixir that will ultimately cure her. Trials hinder her attempts to find it. She's committed to a psychiatric facility. Or she becomes a professional mental patient, a victim of the psychiatric industrial complex. Of course she triumphs, ending up in the light, elixir in hand: accepting medication or getting off medication; finding true love or God; discovering her illness was physical (thank goodness!), not mental after all; devoting herself to meditation or some other supposedly natural remedy; or finding a brilliant physician or freethinking therapist who saves her. On the book's final pages, she's no longer ill or has embraced her illness. She's rejected her diagnosis or accepted it.

My path wasn't that clear. I went to a good university and may or may not have shown promise. I wasn't a professional mental patient. I wasn't a victim. Doctors didn't find a physical cause. Many elixirs were tried: food, alcohol, exercise, various therapies, "natural" remedies, and, finally, psychotropic drugs. The result was pain, monotony, confusion, and messiness.

Yes, I was told—with certainty, one after another—I had anorexia, major depressive disorder (MDD), anxiety disorder, attention deficit hyperactivity disorder (ADHD), obsessive-compulsive disorder (OCD), bipolar disorder. Yes, I almost died.

But I was a willing participant. No one brainwashed me. I believed in and accepted those six diagnoses—adopted them, thought in terms of them, identified myself *as* them, medicalizing my difficulties and discomforts, pathologizing my emotions and thoughts and behaviors.

Embracing a diagnosis can be a good thing. It can increase the likelihood that a person will get help. It can lead someone to find a community of people who suffer from the same diagnosis.[1] It can empower a person.

But it led me into a spiral. Each diagnosis was a self-fulfilling prophecy. The sicker I believed myself to be, the more evidence I found confirming I was sick. The more evidence I had, the more certain I became. The more certain I became, the more willing I was to undergo treatments. The more treatments I underwent, the sicker I believed myself to be.

———

It's too easy to lay blame, but I do. I blame a book: the *Diagnostic and Statistical Manual of Mental Disorders* (DSM).

How can I blame pages, words, letters? Dots. Dashes. Lines. Marks on paper.

Because the DSM is powerful. Jeffrey Lieberman, former president of the American Psychiatric Association (APA), called it "the most influential book written in the past century." Sociologist Allan Horwitz, author of *DSM: A History of Psychiatry's Bible*, writes that it controls the diagnoses we receive and how we think about them.[2]

Which might be fine if the DSM had scientific merit.[3]

Which it doesn't.

Some of the most prominent psychiatrists have referred to DSM diagnoses as constructs and placeholders.[4] Others have admitted that they have no reality, pathologize normality, or are made up. As former National Institute of Mental Health director Thomas Insel put it, we "actually believe [diagnoses] are real. But there's no reality."[5] Allen Frances, one-time chair of the DSM-IV task force, is quoted as saying that DSM diagnoses confuse "mental disorder with the everyday sadness, anxiety, grief, disappointments, and stress responses that are an inescapable part of the human condition."[6] Steve Hyman, another former NIMH director, called DSM diagnoses "fictive categories"[7] and the DSM "an absolute scientific nightmare."[8]

But I didn't know DSM diagnoses were invented and had no validity and little reliability until it was almost too late. Validity, which is considered the most fundamental principle in medicine, would mean that DSM diagnoses can be objectively measured, which they can't.[9] Reliability assumes that multiple clinicians presented with the same patient can rely on the symptoms listed in the DSM and will consistently agree on the patient's diagnosis, which they can't.[10]

It's tempting to fault the DSM's authors, those members of the APA who wielded those words and punctuation marks. How else did so many unproven diagnoses end up on the most recent edition's many, many, many pages? Over the editions, the number of diagnoses and spectrums and subtypes has grown. And grown. The DSM-5 clocks in at 947 pages with 541 diagnostic categories, compared to the scant 132 pages and 128 categories in the DSM-I.[11] The DSM's authors might defend themselves by saying they just want to make sure those who need care receive a diagnosis, even if (they leave this part out) DSM diagnoses are speculative at best.

It's also tempting to reproach the psychiatrists and psychologists and social workers who level DSM diagnoses even though they know those diagnoses are unproven. They claim they *have* to label a patient with a diagnostic code to satisfy the insurance company and to get paid, even if (they leave this part out) it means letting a patient believe she suffers from a diagnosis that's essentially theoretical.[12]

And pharmaceutical companies who have benefited from the DSM's revisions.[13]

And the academic psychiatrists and researchers who have profited from and built their careers on pathologizing normal distress.

But the words—so convincing—do the most damage. They've taken on a life of their own. The DSM has become, as some say, a work of culture.[14] It's socially sanctioned. Many, many people believe it's a scientifically proven medical manual; it's not—not even close.

———

I could be the poster child for the dangers of the DSM. I lived through its most significant editions—the DSMs III, III-R, IV, IV-TR, 5, 5-TR— and received six of its many, many diagnoses. I call them misdiagnoses because all DSM diagnoses are misdiagnoses—i.e., incorrect, inaccurate, inadequate. They were created by loosening criteria, adding specifiers, shifting symptoms, broadening definitions, and lowering thresholds.[15]

How could I have so willingly accepted all those diagnoses and taken all those medications? Why did I believe the words that came from the DSM? I asked so few questions, lived with such little aware-ness. How could I have strayed so far and been so naive?

Like so many who've been diagnosed, I wanted an explanation for what was happening to me—inside me—and no one had warned me about the DSM.

Pathological is everything I wish I'd known. It's an attempt to help others understand the truth about the DSM diagnoses they or their loved ones might receive. All those years, I wasn't the only one being diagnosed. There were the students with autism and oppositional defiant disorder (ODD) I taught in the New York City public schools; Shubi, a young man with schizophrenia found not guilty by reason of insanity for murder; and the many, many college students who came to my office hours and spoke so unquestioningly about their "anxiety disorder" or "depression" or "ADHD brains."

———

I should explain my preoccupation with punctuation. To many people, punctuation is a tedious part of human existence. But I've spent my life writing and reading and teaching people how to write. Punctuation is the basis for communication. It's how we form thoughts. It's the mechanism behind our digital and written interactions, the vehicle that drives our connections and disconnections. Punctuation, like pathology, orders and categorizes; it tries to make sense of what's otherwise disordered.

(When I refer to punctuation, I don't mean to privilege Standard English. Every language and combination of languages and subtype of a language has its own rules: Spanglish, African American Vernacular English, etc. Standard English just happens to be my language.)

Punctuation clarifies. The ancient Greeks put no spaces between words; their ink-laden papyri were a jumble of letters the reader had to decipher: SARAHWOULDNOTEATEVENWHENTHREATENEDWITHHOSPITALIZATION. In the third century BCE, the Greek librarian Aristophanes of Byzantium tried to mediate the madness. He used three dots to separate phrases. Each dot had a position on the line: a dot in the middle of a line—the *komma*—indicated a short pause; one at the bottom—the *kolon*—a medium pause; and one at the top—the *periodos*—a full stop.[16]

———

So many moments in this story call for a full stop, like that day when my mother and I, never finding the psychiatric unit, entered the emergency room. Half full at midday, it lacked urgency. A man rested his elbows on his knees, a plastic bucket at his feet as if waiting for him to vomit. Two children climbed on the seats as a woman called to them to get down.

In the cold of the air-conditioning, we waited for my name to be called. A terrible energy surged through me. Overhead, the fluorescent lights seemed to pulse in time with it.

I was on my sixth diagnosis: bipolar disorder. Already, I'd started to *become* bipolar. Each emotion, every thought, all my behaviors were signs and symptoms of my mental illness. A low mood meant depression; chaotic thoughts and speaking quickly indicated mania.

My name was called. The intake nurse took my blood pressure (normal) and listened to my heart (normal). She had chubby cheeks and a serious but kind demeanor. My temperature was normal, too. I had no physical aches or pains.

After I told her about the darkness and racing thoughts and suicidality, she shifted in her chair and looked at me. Her eyes were tired—exhausted. She said she could admit me to be examined by a psychiatrist.

"And then what?"

She sighed. "You might be transferred to the psychiatric ward here or at another hospital." She paused. "But you don't want that."

I

1

The Weight of a Comma

I t started with a comma. And a cold room. The cold room came first. We waited to be seen by our family doctor at Children's Memorial Hospital. My mom sat on a plastic chair across the room. With her head tipped back resting on the wall, her eyes closed, she took deep breaths, exhaling through pursed lips.

I sat on the examination table, waiting for her to open her eyes. The white paper crinkled beneath me as I pulled my hands from under my thighs and crossed them in front of my chest. Goose bumps covered my forearms, making the thin hairs stand on end. My hospital gown—patterned with childish bubbles though I was about to enter high school—hung loosely below my collarbone. I felt like a child, wanted to be a child, and for my mom to tell me it would all be okay.

Four hours earlier, I'd been on an eighth-grade class trip at Indiana University. The trip might have been a blur except that not eating had made me alert. In one of Indiana's renowned caves, we spelunked in the near-dark. Hunger sharpened my senses. The air was moist against my skin. It smelled of earth and dampness. The drip of distant water echoed in my ears. The weight of my helmet pressed against my forehead. The cave was vivid, dreamlike.

By the third night, it was as if a scrim, like the one that had hung at the back of the stage during our eighth-grade play (*The Hobbit*—I'd debuted as Gollum), hung between me and my classmates. As they lined up for pizza, a light-headedness came over me. My stomach churned though it was empty of food. I took a piece of pizza, let it congeal on my plate, and tossed it in the garbage before the chaperones could see.

The next day, just before we were to leave, that same light-headedness came on. This time, the room spun and my stomach seized. I was going to throw up.

I went to one of the chaperones. She told me to sit. "You need something to settle your stomach." She came back with a soda-fountain Coke in a Styrofoam cup. I brought the cup to my lips. The soda was sweet, bubbly. My stomach did a little flip. Then I leaned over and threw up. She brought me water. I threw that up, too.

On the bus waiting to leave, I balled up my jacket into a pillow and leaned against the window. My stomach was raw, the taste in my mouth putrid. I put on headphones and pressed play on my Walkman. My classmates' voices became muddled. Then they harmonized, then synchronized with the sound of the Eurythmics song piano-keying through my headphones. The bus door suctioned closed. The gears hissed, the engine droned, and we started to move.

An hour and a half later, back at our school, my mom was waiting. She'd been told because she wasn't just my mom; she was the principal. Without a word, she put her hands on my shoulders and looked into my eyes. Her stare was serious. She told me to go wait in the car.

I leaned against our Chevy hatchback and watched as she quickly welcomed back the other students as they filed off the bus. They smiled and waved to the woman they knew as Dr. McCarthy. Her dark skin and short curly hair often made people question if we were related. My sister was dark like her. Blond and light-skinned, I took after my dad.

My mom followed the students into the school and soon came hurrying out. We put my bag in the trunk. In the car, I waited for her to say something. She put the keys in the ignition. I expected her to drive. She stared out the window. I stared at her. Finally, she asked, "What do you think you're doing?"

I didn't have an answer then or when she asked again in the examination room. I was doing what my body told me to do. My stomach hurt. It didn't want food, so I stopped putting food into it. Not eating brought a different kind of ache (dry, empty), but at least it wasn't the sickening, murky pit.

Dr. A came in, his cheeks red and his white hair a little wild. He seemed happy to see us as he went to the sink and washed his hands, chatting with my mom over his shoulder. My mom told him I hadn't eaten in she-didn't-know-how-long.

He pressed the cold stethoscope against my chest. "Take a deep breath," he said. I did, letting it out through pursed lips the way my mom had.

He pointed to the scale. I stepped on. He flicked the weight until it balanced. His cheery expression faded.

I didn't know what it meant to have anorexia nervosa—not in that cold examination room, not in the car on the way home, not in the living room where I sat on the floor smelling the tomato soup and grilled cheese sandwich my dad was making for me in the kitchen. I was only twelve and had grown up sheltered. I attended my mom's school and had fourteen kids in my class. TV was rationed in our house. Magazines weren't yet a part of my world. For my family and most of the general public, the internet didn't exist.

Anorexic.

In the kitchen, my dad and mom whispered. They did that a lot now that they were divorcing. My dad came in with the soup and sandwich on a tray and put it down on the coffee table in front of me. I'd never been allowed to eat in the living room before. Maybe he didn't want me to have to move to the dining room table. Maybe he thought I was that sick. Maybe I was that sick.

I brought a spoonful of soup to my mouth and blew on it through pursed lips. It scared me, that word: *anorexia.* I'd eat. I'd get better. My dad smiled. My stomach churned.

———

The 1980s were the Anorexia Age. Articles on the dangers of dieting appeared in magazines like *Seventeen*. (Ironically, articles on how to diet had been a mainstay of that magazine since 1948.[1]) The well-worn genre known as the eating-disorder memoir was in its heyday.

Journalists called anorexia an "epidemic" though it was reported as affecting fewer than 1 percent of American girls and women.[2] The vast majority were middle to upper class and white, a statistic that often served as a way to trivialize them as starving themselves to death to be fashionably thin.[3]

In anorexia's long history, many have speculated on its nature and causes. The term was coined almost simultaneously by the English physician William Gull and the French neuropsychiatrist Ernst-Charles Lasègue in the nineteenth century.[4] Sigmund Freud—who warned against using psychoanalysis to treat anorexia—and his successors thought it might stem from sexual conflict or a defect of the ego or (I kid you not) the unconscious wish for oral impregnation.[5] Others said it was about control. Or self-punishment. Or the result of disordered family dynamics.[6] Or low self-esteem. Or acting out. Or "the death drive" (the Freudian desire to die).[7] Or a fear of growing up, a way to prevent the full breasts, womanly hips, and fleshy thighs puberty brings. Or vanity, as if bikini season made girls starve themselves until deep crevices formed above their collarbones and each of their ribs could be counted from a distance.[8]

By the time Dr. A christened me with anorexia, it was seen as a complex interplay of factors: cultural (beauty standards for women), psychological (psychoanalytic, family-theory, and social-psychology models), physical (hypothalamic dysfunction, brain lesions), biological (it could be genetic), and historical (shifts in the role that food plays during certain eras).

———

My parents sent me to a therapist. His office was dimly lit. The blinds were always half-closed, letting in faint shafts of sunlight that shone on the wall where his degrees hung.

Dr. S had a beard and wore glasses. Or he didn't. He's hard to re-member. He sat across the room at his desk. I could barely see him behind the stacks of papers and file folders, one of which he took out and glanced through each time I arrived.

It was cold in there, too. The air-conditioning always seemed to be on high. In my seat on the couch, the fan blew directly on me.

That session, like each of our sessions, was long, but I wanted to do well for him and for my parents and to get better. Most of the time, we didn't say much.

He said I was anorexic, too. I wanted to say, *No, I'm not.* I wasn't *Sarah, the anorexic.* Anorexics, he said, dieted; I'd never been on a diet. They weighed themselves; I hadn't been on a scale since the hospital. An-orexia, he said, was characterized by a refusal to eat. I didn't want to eat, didn't want to upset the murky pit in my stomach, and I did eat—a little.

That afternoon, I thought of telling him I wasn't eating because my stomach hurt. But the office was so dark, and he was so far away, be-hind such a large desk and so many stacks of file folders, that I just sat there in the cold and counted the goose bumps on my forearms.

———

I was allowed to stop seeing him when I started high school. The murky pit was practically gone, mainly because the wait was over. Weights had been lifted. I'd started at the competitive high school where my mom wasn't down the hall. I'd had my period, which seemed alien and un-tenable. My parents had separated for good. My sister had gone away to college, so I went back and forth between my dad's new house and my mom's apartment alone.

But my sophomore year the murky pit returned, stronger this time. Heavy. Black. So I starved it again.

I'd been starving it for months the afternoon I sat in English class and tried to pay attention to what Mr. Baker was saying. Mr. Baker: the teacher I idolized. We weren't friendly—strictly teacher-student. He was brilliant and sophisticated, handsome, with a sharp jawline and profoundly blue eyes. He was the first wheelchair user I knew.

In college, he'd been in a car accident while driving a convertible. It flipped over. He'd ended up with a C4 break in his spine, paralyzed from the waist down with restricted use of his upper body. His fingers curved into what's offensively referred to as *claw hands*. Rarely did he write on the board and when he did, he held the chalk precariously in the crook of his thumb. The result was a few scrawled words. He was thin—emaciated, really. Rumor had it that he kept his weight down to alleviate his bedsores.

He treated us like we were smart and could discuss any film or book, even James Joyce's *Ulysses*. He introduced me to F. Scott Fitzgerald's *The Great Gatsby*, a book I loved and read twice in a row, wanting to stay in that strange 1920s flapper world. With him, we learned to analyze books and films as *texts*—finely pieced together, every word thoughtfully chosen, each punctuation mark deliberate.

That afternoon, at the front of the room, he pushed himself toward a TV and VCR that had been moved in so we could watch Orson Welles's *The Lady from Shanghai*. He put in the VHS tape and reminded us to watch for the elements of noir. As the movie played, my stomach contracted, its walls seeming to scrape against each other. I sat up straight but couldn't follow the movie. The main character had or hadn't killed someone. He loved a beautiful woman. She had a husband. At one point, she and the main character talked about suicide but what that had to do with the plot I didn't know. My mind went in circles—arcs of calories, reels of scenes from the movie, swirls of assignments due.

Readjusting my seat, I tried to force myself to focus. It didn't work. Not eating had sapped my energy. All I wanted was to put my head on the table and take a nap. I didn't hunger for his attention; I craved his respect.

The class ended. Mr. Baker reminded us about our tenth-grade term paper. It wasn't due for months, but he recommended we start thinking about it now. The school stressed the paper's importance in our advancement to eleventh grade. If we failed it, we failed the class and might be held back.

I thought of the lunch in my locker: three slim carrot sticks.

Maybe if I hadn't read *The Best Little Girl in the World* over the winter break, things would have turned out differently. The book's 250 pages—which I read quickly and then again and again—were an education.

The novel follows Francesca, a teenager and an anorexic. She renames herself Kessa to signify her transformation into someone thin and in control and stops eating until she ends up in the hospital with a tube in her throat and being force-fed.

On my second and third reads, I skipped the ending, wanting only to know about Kessa. We seemed so much alike. She was white and upper middle class. She got straight A's. She liked the objects on her desk arranged *just so*. There were obvious differences. Kessa lives in Manhattan; I lived in Chicago. She hopes that by being thin she'll gain the approval of her ballet teacher; I played field hockey and my coach couldn't have cared less if I had a long neck and swan arms. Kessa competes with the models in the magazines she collects; I never read fashion magazines. Kessa wants to be clean and unsullied by food, to win a game of her own making in which "thinner's the winner." Unlike her, I didn't feel dirty when I ate and wasn't in competition with anyone. She said nothing about a murky pit in her stomach.

Steven Levenkron's *The Best Little Girl in the World* (1978) is the anorexia urtext. It long predates pro-anorexia websites and thinspiration hashtags that teach girls and women to be "an anorexic."[9] Like the many eating-disorder memoirs published after it, *The Best Little Girl in the World* was more instructional manual and cheat sheet than literature.

Levenkron was a psychotherapist who, after becoming famous as a result of the novel's success, treated singer and drummer Karen Carpenter. Carpenter was the first celebrity anorexic. As half of the musical duo the Carpenters, she, along with her brother, Richard, sold over 90 million records and won three Grammy Awards. Karen, always in the public eye, was the focus of journalists, especially her appearance. A 1975 review of a Carpenters concert in Las Vegas reported that she looked "terribly thin, almost a wraith."[10] (It also criticized her for not having worn a more "becoming" gown.) Anorexia fatalities are often the result of cardiovascular complications like bradycardia, an abnormal slowness of the heart, and heart failure due to starvation. Another estimated 20 percent of anorexics attempt suicide. Carpenter died of heart failure as a result of poisoning from ipecac, a drug that induces vomiting.[11]

According to Randy Schmidt's biography of Carpenter, Levenkron supposedly let her family believe he was a licensed physician. They called him Dr. Levenkron. In reality, he was a therapist who'd written a novel called *The Best Little Girl in the World*, which had been named a Best Book for Young Adults by the American Library Association and was turned into a TV movie, all of which somehow made him an authority on anorexia.

I'd like to think he wasn't to blame for her death or, if he was, that the novel is part mea culpa, part redemption story. It's Levenkron's roman à clef. The novel's other main character, therapist Sandy Sherman, is a thinly veiled version of himself. After Kessa ends up in the hospital with a catheter in her jugular vein that provides her with nutrients, Sherman saves her from herself. Kessa might be seen as the Karen Carpenter Levenkron wished he could have saved, except he published the novel five years before Carpenter's death. The book is an exercise in authorial narcissism. By the end, the focus switches so heavily onto Sherman-as-savior that he replaces Kessa as the novel's hero.

At the time, I barely noticed Sherman, only Kessa. I studied her. She taught me how to think: *My flesh is revolting, my ribs have to jut out, food is the enemy.*

———

I started to count calories, attaching numbers to apple slices and tallying them in a journal. Weighing myself became routine. I smiled at the scale as the numbers went down. I became nimble in my ability to shift food around my plate to make it appear half-empty.

At dinner one night, I chewed and spit the broccoli my mother had served into my napkin. The scalloped potatoes were already well hidden under the pork chop. I deftly leaned over and stuffed the napkin into the cuffs of my jeans. After we cleared the table, I went to the bathroom and flushed the broccoli down the toilet.

Kessa taught me to lie about my weight and what I'd eaten. Like her, I hid my emaciated body under sweatshirts and pajama pants. We differed only in that she quit ballet, and I stayed on the field hockey team, running miles and doing wind sprints even after my weight hovered near a hundred pounds.

One night, my mother and I sat at the dining room table having dinner.

"Eat your chicken," she said.

I wouldn't.

"The potato, then."

I shook my head.

Her response was equally logical. "Fine," she said, standing up. "You'll sit there until you do."

I listened as she washed the dishes in the kitchen—pots clanging, plates clanking, the dishwasher opening and closing. This wasn't just like a scene out of *The Best Little Girl in the World*; it *was* a scene from it. Kessa, too, had been forced to stay at the table until she finished her dinner.

A click and the kitchen light went off. My mom's footsteps on the stairs were followed by the sound of her door closing.

The dining room light seemed dim. The murky pit in my stomach grew. I didn't want to upset my mom, not then and not on the nights when she came into my room and sat on the edge of my bed and told me about the damage I was doing to my body. It wasn't for attention; I'd much rather have been left alone to eat as little as I pleased.

Whereas Kessa retreated and isolated, I had friends and even a boyfriend. Doug was sweet with dark hair and a Roman nose. He was that rare breed: the well-adjusted teenager—all A's, captain of the tennis team. He got along with my parents; he even got along with *his* parents.

But Kessa was my true companion. One afternoon, I stood in front of the hallway mirror and lifted my shirt. The skin on my ribs hung loose. My mom walked up behind me. I pulled the skin away from my jutting ribs. Proof: fat, right there between my fingers. The mind believes what it's told; for months, I'd been telling mine that I was fat.

"See?" I asked.

––––––

Anorexia is from the Greek for "the negation of appetite," but calorie restriction and a preoccupation with weight are only a small part of it.[12] Body dysmorphia—an obsession with a perceived bodily flaw—is its core. My delusions, my insistence that my emaciated body was "fat," confirmed that I was *Sarah, an anorexic*.

Without body dysmorphia, my eating habits might have been considered fasting. A proponent of the fasting craze would have commended me for trying to produce a feeling of well-being, even euphoria. Though some studies find that fasting increases irritability and other "biological symptoms of depression," fasters swear by hunger's positive effects on the brain.[13] They would have told me that ghrelin, the "hunger hormone," which is touted as a potential treatment for major depressive disorder, was helping my mood.[14] If it had been 2020 instead of 1988, and I was, say, male and the CEO of a major tech company, my ability to refuse food for days or a week at a time would have been praised as proof of my strength and discipline.

But there's a difference between fasting and sustained starvation. And I was a teenager. And my hair was falling out in clumps.

––––––

During a tenth-grade class trip—this one for seven days in Minnesota—my diet consisted of a handful of trail mix each day. One evening, after hiking and trust-falling, I stayed in the tent while the rest of my classmates grilled hamburgers and hot dogs for dinner. The smell of charred meat coming from the barbecues outside didn't make me hungry so much as tired.

As I lay on my sleeping bag staring at the tent's thin walls, a soft light filtered in. The sun hadn't even begun to set. To the sounds of cicadas and laughing in the distance, I fell asleep.

When we got back to Chicago, my dad, not my mom, picked me up. He hadn't been called or warned. No one had noticed I hadn't eaten.

The next morning, under the pretense of "going shopping"—something we rarely did—my mom and I headed downtown in a cab. The cab headed east and eventually pulled up in front of a circular building that was part of Northwestern Memorial Hospital. My mother paid the fare. We got out of the cab. On the way up the escalator, we didn't speak.

We entered the eating disorders unit. The waiting room's walls were painted a deep blue. The fabric of the chairs frayed at the edges. I imagined how many other girls had sat there.

Eventually, a nurse called my name. In the examination room, she told me to undress and put on a gown. I did. She directed me to step on the scale: ninety-two pounds. Then she took "my labs"—blood tests, heart rate, blood pressure.

The therapist, a young man in his thirties, reminded me of Sherman from *The Best Little Girl in the World*. So unlike Dr. S, he seemed interested. I asked if he'd be my doctor. He smiled and said no.

As my mom and I waited, we both stared straight ahead at the blue wall. The assistant director of the eating disorders unit called us into her office. She wore her hair twisted in a banana bun and was very thin. We sat in the two chairs opposite her desk.

The assistant director said I'd be admitted to the intensive outpatient program. This wasn't, I learned, good news. It was like being put on probation. I'd be at the hospital four days a week after school for individual and family therapy sessions and meetings with a nutritionist. (No medications—few anorexics were treated with psychotropic drugs back then.) She warned that only one thing would keep me out of the hospital: my lab results. My potassium, electrolyte levels, and blood pressure—all of which could drop dangerously low if I continued to behave the way I was—had to remain stable.

———

Self-denial takes many forms. In the seventeenth century, it was defined as the opposite of self-love.[15] Some say it's about patience, others control. It can be punishing. To some, it's virtuous, an act of renunciation. In religion, it arises out of the desire to find salvation or be redeemed or serve others. It's about faith or spiritual reflection. Or asceticism. Or a monkish devotion to abstinence. Or the piety that drives the devout to abstain out of a love for God.

Sometimes, it's touted as an achievement. Pop psychologists and sociologists have long reported (incorrectly) that self-denial in childhood makes us more successful as adults. It doesn't. The oft-cited 1990 Stanford marshmallow study supposedly showed that if you promised a child a second marshmallow if they waited fifteen minutes before eating the first and the child waited, they would excel in life. The study was flawed. A 2018 experiment that attempted to replicate it found instead that the correlation between self-denial and success vanished almost entirely once researchers controlled for socioeconomic status.[16]

Our views of self-denial are sexist. It's powerful when a man does it, irrational and shallow when a woman does. But it is powerful—even to a sixteen-year-old girl.

———

My psychologist, Laura, had short black hair that curled around her chin. Sitting in a chair beside her desk, I pictured her in high school—an A student, not popular but well-liked.

Light from the window streamed in as she asked about my "anorectic behavior." Was I spitting out my food or measuring my calves or considering taping batteries between my thighs on weigh days? I took these as suggestions and treated them like homework assignments.

It started to feel like a game—except it wasn't. My nails were brittle, my skin dry and cakey. My energy was sapped from not eating. I'd sit in class, my eyes drooping, and try not to fall asleep. My grades had started to slip and then plummet. When I studied, my books seemed gauzy, the words on their pages remote.

She asked how I was doing in school.

"Good," I said. "Good."

————

To confirm my diagnosis, Laura would have flipped through the pages of the DSM-III. As one of the original diagnoses to appear in the DSM-I, anorexia was first described as a psychophysiologic gastrointestinal reaction to stress.[17] Over its many editions, the DSM added subtypes and new food-related behaviors to create an "eating disorders spectrum" that allowed more people to receive a diagnosis. The DSMs III and III-R adopted bulimia nervosa (binging and purging). The DSMs IV and IV-TR added the subtype *eating disorder not otherwise specified* (EDNOS). The DSM-5 made eating disorders a separate chapter (*feeding and eating disorders*), removed EDNOS, and added a bounty of subtypes: *rumination disorder, avoidant/restrictive food intake disorder, other specified eating or feeding disorder, unspecified eating or feeding disorder*, and the dubious *binge eating disorder*.

Laura and I were in the DSM-III era. Psychiatry was supposedly on its way to being a respected field of medicine. Laura would have been confident in the DSM's claims.[18] She might not have known its diagnoses were only more reliable than they'd been in previous editions—which was almost not at all—and that clinicians had complained the diagnostic criteria were unwieldy and arbitrary and didn't apply to patients in the real world.

As diagnoses go, anorexia was a pretty safe bet. It's hard to deny. It's so physical, so visible: my skeletal body, my sharp cheekbones, the peach fuzz covering my abdomen.

————

Time seemed to drag but also to speed by. Some mornings, I woke and washed my face and started to dress for school only to realize that most of the semester had passed. The due date for my tenth-grade term paper was weeks away and then a week away and then a handful of days.

I couldn't even make it through the assigned text: Fyodor Dostoyevsky's *Crime and Punishment*. As I lay on my bed reading the novel, the words blurred on the page. Scene after scene unfolded. The characters rambled on about I didn't know what.

A classmate told me it was about an antisocial, impoverished ex-student, Raskolnikov, who robs and kills an old woman and her sister with an ax and has an existential breakdown as he deliberates whether he should regret what he's done. By the end, his self-justification falls apart, religion sparks a reawakening, and he sees the pointlessness of his crime.

"Right," I said.

I turned one of the final pages and stopped. The skin on the back of my right hand was dry and cracked. Blood seeped from my knuckles. Startled, I sat up. The room seemed to fall away. Everything went black.

Writing the paper didn't go well either. I tried to analyze the imagery, but my thoughts chased each other in circles. I didn't know what I was saying. On the screen of our family computer—a clunky, beige Macintosh Plus—was a jumble of words and punctuation.

———

A week later, the assistant dean pulled me from history class and told me Mr. Baker wanted to see me. I walked through the empty hallways toward his office. At my last visit to the eating disorders unit, I hadn't gained much weight and although my potassium level remained steady, my blood pressure was very low.

I reached Mr. Baker's office and knocked on the open door. He was in his wheelchair at his desk with his back to me. The windowless office he shared with another teacher barely fit two desks and two chairs. I sat in the chair beside him. He adjusted his thin legs and handed me my paper.

I skipped to the last page. In the middle was scrawled an *F* in red pen. The litany of errors he'd written was long: the absence of topic sentences, lack of a clear argument, etc. He said I seemed not to know what the book was about.

"And then," he said, an exasperated expression coming over his face, "there's the way you use commas." He shook his head, dismayed. "Like you're decorating a Christmas tree."

He said I could rewrite the paper. "But it better be good."

I reread *Crime and Punishment*, and I ate. Little bits at a time. Crackers. A slice of cheese. A baked potato. My stomach cramped and ached from being stretched.

The novel was still hard to follow. The Russian names sounded too similar or too foreign to take in, but I managed to understand it well enough to write about the deterioration of Raskolnikov's mind. I typed and typed, trying to describe his mental tirades and how he makes himself ill by tormenting himself with circular arguments about what he's done.

All that was left were commas. I'd barely thought of commas. They joined something and split something else but who knew why. My grammar book was like a foreign language: *subjunctive clauses, appositives, summative modifiers*. Until then, my approach had been to wing it: a dot here, a dash there. It only had to *sound* right.

———

I didn't know it then, but the comma was punctuating my life as an anorexic. It separated items in the list of ways I was falling apart: *dry skin, brittle nails, difficulty concentrating, exhaustion*. It set off information I deemed unimportant: *My symptoms, which included muscle weakness and fainting, were severe*. It coordinated adjectives that described me: *the thin, depressed girl*. It marked an introductory phrase: *Once upon a time, there was a very thin girl*. It created dependent relationships: *Although my family tried to help, I kept getting worse*. It connected independent clauses: *I got worse, and my family was worried*.

The comma didn't always look as it does today. In Aristophanes of Byzantium's three-dot system, the middle dot, which became the comma, indicated the briefest pause, just long enough to take a breath, where the sentence was incomplete. In the late fifteenth century, the Italian scholar and publisher Aldus Manutius gave us the low-hanging, semicircular shape we now have. Some say he lowered the slash, which had been used to separate words; others say he put a tail on the period.

Either way, people eventually started to use it incorrectly as a way "to pause." Not so. That's true for the reader but not the writer. Each person might pause at a different moment when writing a sentence.

I didn't understand the comma's importance—how it clarifies and connects—so I'd used it incorrectly. In my appositive (*Sarah, an anorexic*), I'd formed irrational lists of *target weights, calorie limits, glasses of water to fill my empty stomach*. I joined thoughts that didn't belong together: clauses illogically linked (*I'm hungry, but I shouldn't eat*) and irrational ideas subordinated (*If that bite of toast touches my lips, I'll gain fifty pounds*).

———

The weekend after I turned in the paper, my friend Ryan, a junior, called me at home and said he had a present for me. He was round-faced and sociable, one of those people who was friends with everyone. He drove over in his parents' car.

Once I was in the passenger seat, he handed me a cardboard box. Inside was a kitten, a Siamese tortoiseshell point with mottled beige and brown fur and soft blue eyes. She let out a high-pitched, sweet *mer-ow*.

My mom wasn't pleased. We already had two cats I didn't feed and clean up after. But she didn't make me go back out to the car and give the kitten back. I named the kitten Cappy. She fit in my two hands with just her tail hanging over. That night, she slept in the crook of my neck where she could feel my heartbeat—steady and slow.

That Monday in class, Mr. Baker handed me my paper. I don't remember the grade, but it was decent and I was flagged to go on to eleventh grade. In his comments, he thanked me for my "diurnal and nocturnal efforts." I had to look up both words. He meant he could tell how hard I'd worked on it—day and night. More than that, he said, I'd used commas "mostly right."

———

Summer came. One afternoon, I sat alone in a booth in Mitchell's, a diner-ish restaurant near my high school. It was relatively empty of customers. The waitress stood at my table and scribbled my order of a grilled blueberry muffin (the house specialty) on her order pad. I handed her the plastic-encased menu. She smiled and started to walk toward the kitchen.

To her, I might have been any teenage girl having a sweet treat. A normal girl. A girl who ate what she wanted and didn't obsess about food and her body.

But my mind was still in a loop: the grill, the liquid butter, the muffin, the calories, the fat.

The Best Little Girl in the World offered me a way in but no way out. Kessa's descent into anorexia is clearly plotted, her ascent out of anorexia less so. Recovery occupies a scant thirty-five of the book's 250 pages. Sherman, the heroic therapist, "saves" her by getting her to open up to him about her feelings. He sits with her while she eats, allowing him to observe her compulsive behaviors and rituals around food: cutting her piece of toast into halves and then quarters and only eating a quarter; tapping her fingers on the side of her chair and silently chanting her name to four syllabic beats, four being the "magic number" that would keep her from gaining weight. In the end, it's still unclear whether she'll end up in the hospital again.

After a while, the waitress came over and put down the plate with the blueberry muffin in front of me. I imagined how one of the cooks had sliced it in half, slabbed liquid butter on it, and placed it on the grill. She asked if I needed anything else. I started to cry and hurriedly shook my head.

The muffin lay on the plate, in half, each grilled side oozing butter. I picked up my knife and fork and, like Kessa, cut the muffin into halves and then quarters. Slowly, I took a bite.

〜

2

Consider the Colon

My boyfriend, Chris, went out to the vegetable garden in our backyard and returned with two armfuls of freshly picked yellow squash. "They're going to go bad," he said with a smile and set to work in the kitchen.

The apartment we shared was perfect: a two-bedroom in a two-flat in a not-quite-gentrified neighborhood in Chicago. No one lived in the apartment upstairs. It was like having our own little house. The wood floors were beat up, and the shabby windows drafted frigid air in the winters, but it had a big kitchen, a dining room, and what seemed to us like a huge backyard. Our lives revolved around food-related areas: the kitchen, where Chris cooked; the dining room, where we had dinners with friends; and the garden.

It was his idea to grow vegetables. The garden bordered an abandoned lot on one side and an alley on the other. Only a barbwire fence protected the garden from the cars that sped past, kicking up gravel and dirt and trash. We were so proud of it. In part, it was a response to the limited options for groceries. The local grocery store sold aisles upon aisles of canned food, ten-pound portions of frozen chuck roast, and wilting iceberg lettuce that was often out of stock. We answered with plentiful harvests of zucchini, thyme, and cilantro. Too much basil and too many tomatoes meant we ate balsamic-tomato-basil salads for days in a row. Chicago had its first Whole Foods but compared to our homegrown peppers, theirs looked almost artificial in the glare of the store's fluorescent lights.

That afternoon, while Chris cooked the yellow squash, I took a bath. Our deep claw-foot tub wasn't perfect. Scratches flecked its porcelain finish. One of the lion's feet had broken off and been replaced by an iron stub and wood chips to level it. But the baths it gave enveloped and warmed me.

I wasn't cold anymore, and I'd stopped starving myself. It had happened slowly, taking almost a decade. My freshman year in college, I fell into that strange limbo of eating just enough junk food to keep me bloated and not exactly thin—not eating all day and then giving in to cravings for salty chips and sugary cookies. I'd throw in a sandwich or a salad to make it look like a meal. Disordered eating, maybe, but nothing the eating disorders unit would have taken notice of.

Becoming a Women's Studies major gave me a deeper sense of myself. I wrote essays on the male gaze and protested violence against women in Take Back the Night marches. My brain teemed with thoughts of misogyny and internalized sexism and gender performativity. I learned how the patriarchy and big business and advertising and the media make women believe we were put on this earth to buy uncomfortable lingerie and "trap" men into marriage. I shaved my head—my long, light-brown hair that once reached the middle of my back became stubble. During the late shifts I worked at the campus deli, the drunk frat boys who'd once come in and hit on me (always in a creepy, taunting way) now seemed not to notice me. I was, in my unfemininity, invisible to them—and it was a relief.

Then I read Joan Jacobs Brumberg's *Fasting Girls*, and my relationship to food and my body shifted. Brumberg wrote about women who retreated from society and denied themselves food as acts of defiance and assertions of their rights. During the Middle Ages, women like Catherine of Siena, Margery Kempe, and Julian of Norwich voluntarily emaciated themselves, their hunger making them so weak they hallucinated that God and/or Jesus visited them. The public saw them as mystics or saints, many going to them to be blessed, which undermined and angered the priesthood. After the Reformation, "miraculous maids" put their starvation on display to earn a living at a time when women had no economic rights. People paid to see them. It was the same in Victorian England, when "fasting girls" became a sensation in the press. Brumberg stressed the difference between voluntary fasting for a purpose and anorexia. The book changed how I saw what I'd been doing. Those women were radical; I was senseless.

It helped that the eating disorders unit was far away. No one was around to remind me that I had anorexia. No longer defined by my *-ia*, no longer thinking in the appositive (*Sarah, the anorexic*), I stopped believing I was one.

While in the bath, I left the door open so I could hear Chris chop onions and click the burners on the stove and run the water in the kitchen sink. Cappy came in, *mer-ow*ed, rubbed against the tub, and walked out. I didn't ask Chris what kind of soup he was making out of all that squash. I'd eat what was given.

His relationship with food was one of devotion. When he cooked, each cube of bouillon, every clove of garlic, deserved respect. He ate healthy meals, usually stopped when he was full, and didn't manipulate or fear food the way I had. On our days off, he'd cook all afternoon, making big batches of potato leek or white bean and fennel soup. Soup was the staple of our diet, mainly because it was cheap.

I finished my bath and dressed and sat on the couch to read. Our life together was simple. We had no internet. The TV stayed in the closet and was only brought out to watch the occasional show. We worked nights in the service industry—he as a bartender, I as a server. During the day and on our nights off, he wrote songs and performed with an avant-garde theater company on the South Side and I wrote strange, ethereal short stories no one read.

In our social circles, without social media, we didn't hunger for money and fame. It was the 1990s. Being "indie" was still possible, not watered down by the flatness of the internet, where all albums—major or indie, well funded or on a shoestring—look the same. To Chris, the pinnacle of success was to be signed to the indie record label Thrill Jockey—which produced bands like The Sea and Cake and Tortoise. I thought only of writing, not about getting published, and knew nothing about MFA programs and agents. We just wanted the next day to be as good as the one before.

There was a sense of plenty. Rent was affordable. Our furniture and clothes were almost all secondhand. We didn't buy *stuff*. Most of our money went to CDs and books, under-ten-dollars bottles of wine, groceries, and food and catnip for Cappy.

Chris called me to the kitchen. On the table sat two steaming bowls of pureed yellow squash soup. It didn't matter that it was warm out. We sat kitty-corner to each other.

Seven years older than I was, he was genuine and cool and talented and funny. My family loved him—my mother, my father, my stepmother, my sister, my brother-in-law—and his love for me was palpable. I'd never had anyone give of themselves the way Chris did. Early in our relationship, after finishing a solo hiking trip of a section of the Appalachian Trail, he drove his VW Bus all night to be with me as soon as he could.

He lifted his spoon and blew on his soup to cool it. I put my hand on his free hand and gently squeezed. He lowered his spoon to the bowl and wove his fingers through mine.

"Thank you," I said, my eyes tearing up.

He tilted his head, clearly surprised by the emotion squash soup had evoked in me. "You're welcome."

I raised our joined hands to my lips and kissed the back of his hand. So much had changed. I was cured.

———

The word *cure* doesn't mean what we think it means. The primary definition is "to take care of." In that sense, I was "cured." I'd learned to take care of myself. What we think of when we read the word *cure* is the secondary definition that appears in the *Oxford English Dictionary*:

someone being healed from a disease. It first appeared in Wycliffe's Bible in reference to physical diseases. It wasn't until the sixteenth, seventeenth, and eighteenth centuries that we started to believe in cures for emotions like love, grief, and desire.

If I'd asked Laura if I was cured, she'd have said no, citing the statistics on anorexia. There was a good chance I'd relapse. The "anorectic behavior" would start again. I'd develop bradycardia and die of heart failure due to starvation. Or I'd die by suicide. Most likely, alcoholism was in my future, and that could lead to death, too.

I'd have told her she was wrong; I wasn't *Sarah, the anorexic*, anymore. I ate the soups Chris made, heavy on olive oil and finished with butter; indulged in one bowl (sometimes two) of ice cream in his presence, never in secret; and dined out on rich meals of fatty salmon and creamy mashed potatoes. It could all be indexed: a balanced diet, unrestricted calories, normal weight, no preoccupation with thinness, no scale in the house. I practically celebrated food with friends—mostly Chris's. (I'd never needed a lot of friends.) At our dinner parties, I ate apple-pecan arugula salad, baked cod with sour cream and dill, and figs with chocolate for dessert. I could pay attention to the conversation and not count calories. The ratio of my healthy thoughts and actions to my unhealthy ones was ten to one (10:1), maybe twenty to one (20:1).

But the prevailing view is that most DSM diagnoses are chronic.[1] People with them can "experience relief." They can "manage." They can even live "a satisfying life."[2] But they can't be cured.

———

One afternoon on my way to work, I stopped at the used bookstore. M.F.K. Fisher's *The Gastronomical Me* stood on the shelf, facing out. On the cover was a black-and-white photograph of Fisher wearing dark lipstick with her hair swept back in a bun, a chopstick holding it in place (exactly how I wore my hair). Fisher stared at the camera—bold, ready. I'd never heard of her and didn't know that she defined the

American tradition of food writing as a mix of memoir, how-to guide, and adventure story. The book was a chronicle of her life as a woman with an unapologetically voracious appetite.

I read the foreword. She wrote that food is one of our three basic needs, along with security and love. The three were "so mixed and mingled and entwined that we cannot straightly think of one without the others." Her adoration of food was methodical and nostalgic. I flipped through the book, stopping to read her description of eating an oyster in all its slick, briny distinctiveness; her reflection on dining practices in ancient Egypt and the love of yogurt and honey among the ancient Greeks; and her remembrance of how she kept the "wolf" of hunger at bay amid rations and food shortages during World War II.

That night I sat with my coworkers at the bar folding napkins for the night's service. Half of them were artists or aspiring actors who waited tables to pay their rent. Napkins folded, we polished the glasses and silverware and sampled the night's special: skate wing in a beurre blanc sauce. My favorite: rich, buttery, the fish flaky but moist. No flicker of panic passed through me as it melted onto my tongue.

The restaurant was "cool." With no street sign to indicate the entrance, you had to be in the know, which meant that annoyed and sometimes irate suburban patrons often arrived late for their reservations. There, food wasn't just eaten; it was studied. The chef had taught me the nuances among filet mignon, Chateaubriand steak, and beef Wellington. I learned the difference between a broth and consommé, crudités and charcuterie, a tart and a galette.

Before service started, I stood by the kitchen window and chatted with one of the line cooks. Their shifts started in the early afternoon and, after standing in front of a hot stove for six or eight or ten hours, ended whenever they'd broken down the kitchen for the night. And all for a fraction of what we made working a fraction of the time. Service, for them, was pressured and dangerous, given the sharpness of the knives and the extreme heat of the pans. The line cook hitched up the sleeve of his chef's coat. Burn marks striped his forearms. *Food*, I thought. *He'd done that for the love of food.*

A four-top was seated in my section. I took their order, brought their wine, and opened it at the table. At the kitchen window, a server joked about a British couple who'd complained about their entrées the night before. "Like they have any right to talk about food. What have they given the world? Shepherd's pie?"

I laughed. Then a sick feeling came over me. Heavy sick. Was the murky pit back? No, the skate wing must have been too rich.

The sick feeling was soon accompanied by a burning sensation. It got worse. And worse. After half an hour, I went to my manager and asked to be cut. He hedged, worried it would get too busy. Eventually, he gave in.

By the time I got home, the burning was intense. I kneeled between the toilet and tub and waited to throw up.

––––––––

The stomachaches that followed were different. The murky pit was re-placed by bloating and nausea and fullness and burning pain. Not eat-ing made it worse, not better. All I wanted was to eat. My thoughts of food were hopeful and desperate, but all I could stomach was steamed spinach or vegetable soup or dry toast—and often not even those.

In the late afternoons, the nausea and burning were accompanied by surges of a terrible energy that rushed through my chest and made me feel on edge. The edginess exhausted me, but my racing thoughts and pounding heart, which echoed in my ears, kept me up at night. I'd lie next to Chris and stare at the curtain blowing in the breeze coming through the open window.

And then there were the migraines, which came with blinding auras that laid me out for hours at a time. A single dot on my field of vision would tendril out into flashes of light. I'd draw the shades and lie down in the bedroom. These headaches left me in a fog that made reading and writing seem impossible.

Pregnancy was ruled out. I wasn't sent for a brain scan because I'd always had migraines, just not that blinding. My primary care physician sent me for a colonoscopy that showed my small and large intestines were fine. A barium swallow showed a possible ulcer but not severe enough to cause the pain I described.

Soon, I was regularly asking to be cut at work. Then I started to call in sick, something I never did. Finally, I asked my manager to schedule me for two shifts a week, which didn't help our finances.

I spent a lot of time waiting for Chris to come home. One night, I pulled out the TV and turned to the public television channel. A black-and-white movie was on. I settled onto the couch. Cappy hopped up and nestled in my lap.

It was a Humphrey Bogart and Lauren Bacall movie I didn't catch the name of. In it, Bogart is accused of murder and gets plastic surgery to change his identity. In the scene when he removes the bandages to see his new face for the first time, he looks in the mirror and rubs his chin with concern. Bacall says she likes him better. He smiles. He has a new identity, a chance to be free.

I thought I'd been given a new identity. I was finally rid of my appositive, my -*ia*, but now my freedom was being taken away. The colon that once introduced my good health (*I was cured: eating well, getting fresh air, exercising*) now signaled a different set of symptoms (*These problems were new: burning stomachaches, depression, nervousness*).

———

Sometime later, while Chris worked the lunch shift, I went to our bookshelf. William Styron's *Darkness Visible: A Memoir of Madness* wasn't a book I remembered buying. It must have belonged to Chris. The spine was barely creased and the pages crisp.

I sat in our backyard in the sun and finished most of it in one sitting, getting sunburned in the process. My legs felt shaky as I stood. It was as if Styron was speaking directly to me. His depression didn't make him feel heavy and sleep all day; he had what his doctors called atypical depression: fine in the morning—buoyant, even—only to be crushed by gloom and dread and anxiety in the late afternoon. I wanted to ask if he'd had a stomachache, too.

Styron gave me my first understanding of depression. He referred to it as a "mood disorder"—which sounded serious—and defined it as a biochemical malfunction that resulted from "systemic stress" amid "neurotransmitters of the brain" that caused the depletion of serotonin. It sounded so scientific. So reliable. So valid.

It was the "age of depression," but I didn't know that.[3] The antidepressant Prozac had been around for nearly a decade and was grossing the pharmaceutical company Eli Lilly $2 billion annually.[4] Elizabeth Wurtzel's depression memoir *Prozac Nation* was a bestseller.

Styron mentions the DSM in passing, referring to it as the "psychiatrists' bible." I'd never heard of it. DSM? He said he studied it the way a medical student would to better understand his "madness." *Madness.*

———

In 1990, when *Darkness Visible* was published, Styron likely would have studied the DSM-III-R (*R* for *revision*). From the way he describes his diagnosis—with certainty—he must have believed the DSM was a work of science.

It's clear he wasn't aware of the damage done first by the DSM-III and then by the III-R. The DSM-III was headed by Columbia University Professor of Psychiatry Robert Spitzer. As task-force leader, Spitzer, who's often referred to as one of the most influential psychiatrists in recent history, transformed our concept of mental disorders through the DSM. Journalist Alix Spiegel sums it up best: Spitzer "took the Diagnostic and Statistical Manual of Mental Disorders . . . and established it as a scientific instrument of enormous power."[5] Spitzer and his coauthors created what looked like a scientific manual,[6] one that would prove psychiatry's standing in medicine, even though many of its diagnoses were based on arbitrary categorizations.[7] The DSM-III-R (*R* for *revision*) was meant to repair inconsistencies in the DSM-III. But Spitzer ended up doing a repeat performance, reordering diagnostic categories and adding twenty-five more—increasing the DSM-I's 128 diagnoses and the DSM-II's 193 and the DSM-III's 228 to 253—based on no new empirical research.

The DSM-III could be seen as having twisted the definition of *disease* (itself a subject of ongoing debate) to make it fit the limited data they had. According to *Taber's Medical Dictionary*, a disease requires not just complaints and symptoms but "laboratory or radiographic findings." A disease is objective, tangible, measurable. The DSM-III offered no such findings but still stated that its diagnoses were marked by signs and symptoms with "an inference that there is a behavioral, psychological, or biological dysfunction."[8] The word *biological* implied the manual's disorders were in some way objective. Although Spitzer said, "There is no assumption that the organismic dysfunction or its negative consequences are of a physical nature," the DSM-III, as medical historian Edward Shorter writes, turned "diagnoses into diseases."[9]

By the time Styron had the DSM in his hands, psychiatry was pushing the brain-disease theory hard. In her influential 1984 book, *The Broken Brain*, psychiatrist and researcher Nancy Andreasen wrote, "The major psychiatric illnesses are diseases. They should be considered medical illnesses just as diabetes, heart disease, and cancer are. The emphasis in this model is on carefully diagnosing each specific illness from which the patient suffers, just as an internist or neurologist would."[10] Others followed: Nobel Laureate Eric Kandel, former NIMH director Thomas Insel, even the National Institutes of Health.[11] Members of the psychiatric community argued over the definition of *disease* in an effort to make mental disorders fit it.[12]

Psychiatry has been trying to make DSM diagnoses into diseases for thirty years, but they haven't been able to—at least not without manipulating meanings and twisting definitions. Disorders like depression and anxiety aren't akin to cancer or diabetes. The comparisons don't hold up. Diseases like cancer and diabetes can be determined using an objective measure; DSM diagnoses were and are entirely subjective. They're based on self-reported symptoms and a clinician's opinion. I tend to be very thirsty, get hungry to the point of extreme irritability and dizziness, get tired, and urinate fairly frequently (TMI, I know), but I don't have diabetes—a blood test would show that. I could never just be told I have diabetes, identify as a diabetic, and start taking insulin. But if I walk into a psychiatrist's office and reveal that I've been known to worry, often can't control the worry, can feel restless and keyed up, often can't concentrate, get irritable, lie awake in the middle of the night, and often avoid social situations, I can be diagnosed with generalized anxiety disorder (GAD) and no objective measure can say otherwise. I'd likely walk out of that psychiatrist's office believing I *have* anxiety disorder, a mental illness, and may start psychotropic medication.

DSM diagnoses weren't—and still aren't—valid. In clinical nosology, a diagnosis is valid if it exhibits "essential properties."[13] DSM diagnoses can't be reified, meaning they don't exist outside of someone observing them.[14] They aren't even discrete disease entities, meaning they aren't clear-cut; diagnoses and symptoms overlap.

The hundreds of new diagnoses that appeared in the DSM-III and III-R were essentially invented and ratified by committee. Spitzer and his coauthors attached symptoms to diagnoses and created diagnoses to fit symptoms. (He supposedly had an unbridled enthusiasm for classifying. Something of a modern-day Linnaeus, Spitzer admitted, "Ever since I was a child, I liked to sort things."[15] He's said to have delighted in clustering symptoms and arranging and rearranging them into theoretical bins to determine which best belonged with which diagnosis.) Allen Frances, who edited the personality disorders section and led the DSM-IV task force, said the DSM-III's creation "wasn't pretty to watch—it had the feel more of virtuoso performance art than scientific deliberation."[16]

Originally, the DSM didn't claim scientific authority. The APA published it to give hospital psychiatrists and clinicians a common language. That language primarily reflected the dominant theory of the age: psychodynamic and psychoanalytic psychiatry.[17] The DSM-I (1952) broadly distinguished among mental disorders. The symptom lists were vague, sometimes ending with "and so forth."[18] Organic brain disorders (like epilepsy) were distinguished from those thought to be the result of external pressures—both psychotic (e.g., schizophrenia) and neurotic (e.g., anxiety and depression). It had little influence and wasn't thought of as a definitive nosology, meaning a medical, scientific classification of diseases.[19]

After the DSM-I, each edition tried to assert more scientific authority. The DSM-II (1968) remained psychodynamic in orientation and expanded definitions of *mental disorders* to include milder conditions that affected more of the general public. With few exceptions, it removed the word *reaction* from its pages.[20] No more *depressive reaction* or *anxiety reaction* or *schizophrenic reaction*; there was simply depression, anxiety, and schizophrenia. Although the DSM-II stated that the removal of *reaction* didn't mean its diagnoses were fixed disease entities, its absence said that the causes of mental disorders, which couldn't be proven, didn't matter as much as the symptoms themselves. The paradigm had started to shift.[21]

The DSM-III (1980) was a turning point.[22] Since then, biological psychiatrists, researchers, drug companies, the Food and Drug Administration (FDA), and the National Institute of Mental Health (NIMH) have wanted a diagnostic classification system that was—or *seemed* to be—based on hard science.[23] The DSM-III-R (1987) maintained the DSM-III's declarations of scientific legitimacy. The DSM-IV (1994) introduced the idea that a diagnosis had to significantly impair the "overall" functioning of a person. What this meant was unclear because no biomarkers existed to define *impairment* and *dysfunction*. The DSM-IV-TR (2000) introduced few changes. Even though neuroscience failed to prove definitively that DSM diagnoses had objective realities, the DSM-5 (2013) said, no, its diagnoses weren't biological but just wait, not to worry, someday the neuro-circuitry in the brain would (likely, maybe, possibly) show that they were.[24] (It seems convenient that psychiatry uses the terms *illness* and *disease* and *disorder* interchangeably, causing the rest of us and the media to do the same.)

We could argue that it doesn't matter; DSM diagnoses are *disorders*, as the title of the manual suggests. Without a test or physical indicator of what constitutes even just one DSM diagnosis, *disorder* is all psychiatry really has—but even that's shaky. As Jerome Wakefield writes, the "claim of psychiatry to be a medical discipline depends on there being genuine mental disorders."[25] The problem is that *disorder* is a value judgment. We can't say what makes a response to a life event "disordered" for every person in every situation. Even if we held to Wakefield's definition of *disorder* as "harmful dysfunction," "harmful" is subjective. Psychiatry doesn't have its own definition of *disorder*. Often it relies on terms like *distress* and *disability*, but those, too, are relative. If, as the DSM authors admit, a *disorder* can't be defined,[26] and the task forces and committees that write the DSM don't have a way to quantify *disorder*, what are we being diagnosed with?

Styron wouldn't have asked this question as he sat at his desk with a light shining down on the pages of the DSM, him taking it in as science, as truth.

———

During a trip to New York, my symptoms were at their worst. The carpeting of our cheap Midtown hotel room was so dingy and threadbare as to be barely beige. The windows looked out onto a brick wall. The sounds of traffic—cars screeching, ambulance and police sirens wailing, horns honking—must have come from the street, but we didn't hear them, not over the din of the window air conditioner's battered fan. The room smelled of the mildewy shower. I should remember the color of the bedspread—should remember more about the hotel room—because I spent a lot of time in it alone.

Mainly, I read while Chris visited friends and went out to eat. My stomach burned and ached. Each afternoon came the crushing dread and terrible surging energy.

As we packed to go home—me on the bed, him putting his clothes in our suitcase—I said I didn't feel well.

"I *know*," he said, more irritated than I'd ever heard him. "I *know* you don't feel well."

I expected this to be followed with something along the lines of *I've had enough* or *I can't take it*. He stopped and reached out his arms to me. As I went to him, I wanted so much to be well and not be the person I was. He held me, my head against his chest, and stroked my hair.

———

The afternoon I had my first suicidal ideation, I sat on our couch with Cappy snuggled in the crook of my arm. Chris was out. Light raindrops ticked against the window behind me.

The stomachaches—now acidic with seizures of nausea—continued. Reading became increasingly difficult, so I started to reread Fisher's books. That afternoon, my eyes drifted over her words, barely taking them in.

It's hard to say if the thought or the image came first. The thought must have: *This is never going to end.* Then came the image: the bathroom, the tub—our claw-foot tub—my body inside the tub, my wrists slit, the bathwater red.

The image stayed too long. I nudged Cappy onto the couch and stood. I paced. It flashed through my mind—again and again—almost in sync with the rain against the window.

Sitting on the edge of a chair at the kitchen table, I started to panic. Was I suicidal? What did *suicidal* even mean? Most of what I knew came from movies, pop culture, and the media. Celebrities had died that way: Ernest Hemingway, Marilyn Monroe, Sylvia Plath, Virginia Woolf, Kurt Cobain. I'd heard most about Cobain, who'd died a few years earlier and whose death was almost always described as "tragic."

Researchers and clinicians still presumed suicidal behavior was a symptom of mood disorders like major depressive disorder (MDD) or borderline personality disorder (BPD).[27] Suicidal behavior disorder hadn't yet been considered a distinct condition.[28]

Not that I would have been aware of that. Depression and the DSM and psychiatry and suicide weren't part of my life. I had one friend who took medication, but we'd never really talked about it. Back then, *mental health* wasn't a buzzword.

When Chris came home, he made us dinner: tomato, fennel, white bean soup and a baguette. I thought of Fisher, who wrote that to nourish oneself demands honesty: "There is food in the bowl, and more often than not, because of what honesty I have, there is nourishment in the heart, to feed the wilder, more insistent hungers."[29] Honesty was a precursor to satiety. Without being honest—with ourselves and with others—we have no hope of feeling full.

After we—he—ate and cleaned up, I sat on the couch. He went into the dining room to practice guitar. Each plunk of the country blues song he played—Robert Johnson and Blind Willie McTell—told me to say it, go in the dining room and sit next to him: *I just imagined my death.* Or go into my writing room and try to explain it in a letter— *Dear Chris: I may be suicidal.*

I went to bed and lay there, staring up at the ceiling, unable to understand it myself.

———

When I first read *Darkness Visible*, I didn't notice how Styron uses colons to introduce and signal what's to come. As a writer, I was ashamed of my ignorance of punctuation's rules and meaning, but it still meant little to me. My how-to-write-fiction and how-to-write-poetry books never mentioned it.

The colon explains his depression—"Its most famous and sinister hallmarks: confusion, failure of mental focus and lapse of memory"— and how, for him, it came on late in the day—"There was now something that resembled bifurcation of mood: lucidity of sorts in the early hours of the day, gathering murk in the afternoon and evening."[30] He uses it to introduce a quote from Camus's famous essay on suicide: "'Judging whether life is or is not worth living amounts to answering the fundamental question of philosophy.'"[31] The colon offers a miserable prognosis for the depressive who has suicidal thoughts: "The argument I put forth was fairly straightforward: the pain of severe depression is quite unimaginable to those who have not suffered it, and it kills in many instances because its anguish can no longer be borne."[32] And lists the many "fallen artists" who've succumbed to suicide: "Hart Crane, Vincent van Gogh, Virginia Woolf, Arshile Gorky, Cesare Pavese, Romain Gary, Vachel Lindsay, Sylvia Plath, Henry de Montherlant, Mark Rothko, John Berryman, Jack London, Ernest Hemingway,

William Inge, Diane Arbus, Tadeusz Borowski, Paul Celan, Anne Sexton, Sergei Esenin, Vladimir Mayakovsky—the list goes on."[33]

Colons don't appear in the strange, ethereal short stories I wrote then. Not knowing how to use them, I just pretended they didn't exist. Never mind the lists and descriptions I could have introduced, the explanations I could have provided, the words I may have defined, the people I might have quoted.

The colon is a holy punctuation mark. Like the comma, it came to us via Aristophanes of Byzantium's three-dot system, but it was put to use in 400 AD when the priest Saint Jerome used it to mark off sections of the Vulgate Bible to be sure monks read the word of God correctly.[34] The colon told the monks to pause longer than the middle dot but not quite as long as the high one. Pacing. Proper reverence for the words they spoke.

It doesn't pace or join or separate or end; it prophesizes. Derived from the Greek word for *limb*, it signals an extension. It appears after a clause, a complete thought (*I wanted only two things: to be with Chris and to write*). Like two headlights, it shines a light on what's to come: lists (*Maybe I could have done more to make myself well: rested, eaten better, exercised*) and information (*Suicidal thoughts are only cause for alarm in one instance: when passive thoughts become active thoughts*).

––––––

I forced myself back to work. One night, I stood at the bar and ordered a bottle of wine for a table. Service had started when the burning in my stomach flared. The weight of dread descended. The terrible surging energy rose in me. They met in the middle of my chest.

The bartender came back and set the bottle of Pinot Noir on the cocktail tray. He asked, "Are you okay?" I didn't answer. At the host station, my manager stood talking to a couple who had eaten in my section. Although their voices were calm and easy, they seemed to crack against my chest.

When the couple finally left, I told my manager I had to leave. His look said, *Are you kidding?* I brought my hand to my forehead. As I did, he stared at it. It was shaking.

I got home to a dark, empty apartment. Still shaking, I sat on the couch, the phone in my hand. Fear—unreasonable and paralyzing—rose in me.

On the couch, I stared at the bathtub. A string of thoughts followed: *This is never going to end. It will never get better. It will only get worse. I can't take this.*

No image came. The thoughts seemed fleeting—just sentences in my mind. Nothing serious.

When Chris got home, I was in bed. Again, I stared at the ceiling. The sound of him opening the fridge reached me. A moment later came the clink of a bottle on the counter, a drawer opening and closing, the fizz of the cap being pried off the bottle, the tap of the cap on the counter. I pictured him going into the living room. Eventually, he'd sit on the couch, headphones on, and listen to music.

I wish I could say I got out of bed and that Chris was on the couch and that it took a minute for him to look up and when he did, I knew I could tell him everything and that I did, that I told him about the image and the thoughts, and that he looked alarmed and because he rarely looked alarmed, his alarm alarmed me and he reached out and drew me to him and I rested my head on his chest. More than anything, I wish I could say he looked in my eyes and asked what we should do and that the *we*—his inclusion of himself in the situation, *my* situation—brought a rush of relief because I wasn't alone.

But I don't remember telling him. I remember wondering what the image and the thoughts meant about me. I remember being scared. I remember wanting to tell him. I remember—at some point—the two of us perched on the edge of the couch, him facing me, his knees touching mine.

3

Suspension Points

The next year and a half is riddled with gaps, ellipses. Ellipsis marks—the dot-dot-dot (. . .) of punctuation—are all about erasing, forgetting, denying. The word *ellipsis* comes from the Greek, meaning "to fall short" or "to leave out." Omissions. Blackouts. Lapses of memory: *We had dinner, drank a bottle of wine, talked about our relationship, ordered another bottle, and then . . .* The failure to recall.

Unlike other punctuation marks that clarify, the ellipsis instills doubt. It marks the inability to finish a thought (aposiopesis): *I drank a lot, but I wasn't sure if I was an alcoholic or . . .* It's a mark of hesitation. Had Chris tried to talk to me about my drinking but held back? Had he stopped out of a wish not to upset me? *Sarah, you really need to . . . Never mind.* Ellipses can signal a lack of self-confidence: *I was . . . doing well.*

Ellipsis points, as we know them, date back to the sixteenth century but didn't come widely into use until the seventeenth and eighteenth centuries. Often, they appeared not as three dots but as multiple hyphens, dashes, or asterisks. One of the earliest recorded uses of ellipses appears in the 1588 edition of the English translation of Roman dramatist Terence's *Andria*.[1] The translator used multiple hyphens to tell the actor when a character trailed off or was interrupted.

Sometimes called suspension points, ellipses can be addicting. (People have been trying to prevent their overuse since the eighteenth century.[2]) Once you start to use them to denote a falling off, an absence, or a dramatic pause, well . . . it's hard to stop.

It's teasing, how they imply more is to come: *There was no way of knowing what would happen next . . .*

————

Seattle wasn't what we expected. We'd moved after visiting the city on a misleadingly sunny weekend. The Puget Sound had glistened in the sunlight, and Mount Rainier stood majestic in the distance. The city seemed to us a bastion of musicians and writers. We'd gone to the Tractor Tavern in Ballard to see a band. While walking down the street in First Hill, checking out possible neighborhoods, we'd passed a woman wearing pajamas and a bathrobe sitting on her front stoop reading. Everyone, it seemed, played music. Everyone, it seemed, read.

We were wrong. Amazon was on the rise, bringing with it not books and readers but exorbitant rents and dot-comers. We lived in a tiny two-room apartment, so different from our place in Chicago. The grunge phenomenon—thanks to Sub Pop Records and Nirvana and Pearl Jam and Soundgarden—had drawn many (too many) aspiring musicians, and Chris wasn't having luck booking gigs. He'd left the service industry and was a baker in a small café. I'd become a sommelier and had little time to write. At least no suicidal images or thoughts had followed me there.

I'd interviewed for a position as a part-time writing tutor at one of Seattle's community colleges but hadn't heard. During my interview, the director of the center had been welcoming. She was one of those women you'd describe as "sharp" but with kind eyes behind her glasses. The writing center seemed heavenly. Extra pens and scrap paper were on all the tables. The fall term hadn't started and no students were there, but it had the same mentally nourishing energy found in libraries. It smelled of the grammar books that lined the shelves.

I pulled out my laptop and sat at the kitchen table to check my email.

I'd had to take a grammar and punctuation proficiency test. As soon as I sat down, the director put the paper in front of me and my hangover kicked in. I hadn't intended to drink the night before, but Chris and I split a bottle of wine and then a second bottle. It had seemed harmless enough—the two of us at our kitchen table, Cappy on the window ledge soaking in the rays of a rare Seattle sunset. But at the writing center, as I tried to fill in sentences with the correct punctuation, my mind turned foggy: *I want the job but, my grammar and punctuation skills might not be strong enough.*

Cappy hopped on my lap. On my laptop were two emails. I opened the one from the director: *I'm happy to inform you . . .*

The first meeting was in two days. This was it: new job, new life. I'd drink less. I couldn't tutor hungover and foggy. I'd get back to writing.

———

That afternoon, I went to work. As I closed the restaurant door behind me, the sound echoed against the dining room's white walls and twenty-foot ceilings. The waitstaff wouldn't be in for hours. On the other side of the frosted glass wall that separated the front of the house from the kitchen, the sous chef and line cooks prepped for the night's service. The tables in the dining room were bare except for the white tablecloths.

No meetings with purveyors were scheduled for that afternoon; I had a study session for my Master Sommelier exam that would be held in Las Vegas in a couple of weeks. I was an accidental sommelier. I'd been waiting tables at the restaurant when they fired the first sommelier for stealing. I was very good at distinguishing between the earthiness of a French Pinot Noir and the dense berry fruit of one from the Willamette Valley. They asked me to fill the position.

Wine excited and interested me in a geeky, knowing-information-no-one-else-cares-about way. One wine might smell so much like the earth that you could practically feel the dirt between your fingers. Another would have such a velvety finish, you felt as though you were eating the richest dark chocolate. Another would pop with raspberry like it came from the actual fruit.

Working in restaurants had been a way to earn money to write. Suddenly, I spent all my time and energy on wine. I was getting media attention because I was young and a woman in a male-dominated industry and Pacific Northwest wines were *it*. I was quoted in *Wine Spectator* and featured in *Fortune* (Chris and I noted the irony, given my meager salary). It seemed right to register for the Master Sommelier exam. My bosses were excited. There seemed no way to quit and back out.

At a table near the window looking out on the street, I placed several wineglasses in front of each of three chairs. I put down a wine bucket to be used as a spittoon. Today—from now on—I'd use it.

There was no need to swallow—ever. A wine's appearance in the glass told a real sommelier what she needed to know. Its aroma revealed 80 percent of the information. One sip, a few swishes in the mouth, and a spit were enough to gauge the balance (alcohol, acidity, tannin, and fruit), intensity (its "body"), and finish (the taste that lingers).

There came a knock on the restaurant door. The two other sommeliers in my study group arrived. We weren't officially sommeliers and should have been called wine directors, but everyone used the title casually back then. They'd already completed the two-day intensive and written-theory portion of the introductory exam and were prepping for the advanced; I was on stage one.

We sat. They uncorked the wines they'd brought (all in wine sleeves to hide the labels). I half listened as they gossiped about other restaurants and discussed the wines they'd added to their lists. I pulled out my notebook and a pen to take notes during the tasting. They already had theirs out.

We raised the first glass of red and searched for signs of visible sediment, analyzed its concentration (pale? medium? deep?), noted its primary colors (purple? ruby? garnet?) and secondary colors (orange tinge or blue?), and assessed its staining and tearing (its "legs," which indicate the alcohol content).

I enjoyed the detective work of guessing a wine. I swirled my glass to release the wine's aroma: jammy fruit, new wood, spice, a hint of earthiness. Easy: American, Cabernet, or a blend. I smelled it again. Napa or Sonoma. Maybe early 1990s.

Sip. Swish . . .

Spit, I told myself as I swallowed.

The buzz of the first sip was always the best. A warm feeling in my belly. A cascade of relief after it was absorbed in my stomach lining and seeped into my bloodstream and spread, eventually blocking the signals between my brain cells, giving me a kind of chemical serenity that stilled my thoughts.

One of my cohorts reached for the wine bucket, brought it close, and spit. I took another sip of my wine. And another.

Alcoholism has been described as a sign of insanity, a moral failing, a social problem, and a disease.[3] During the eighteenth century, psychiatrists referred to alcoholism as *oinomania*, "wine mania." It could be acute, periodic, or chronic. An alcoholic was seen as exhibiting temporary insanity and was often treated in an asylum.[4] During the nineteenth and early twentieth centuries, the temperance movement argued that alcoholism was more of a social problem than one that affected individuals. After World War II, it was categorized as an addiction and a biological disease.

The DSM has primarily generated confusion in its classification of alcoholism as a mental disorder; the DSM authors seem unable to decide if alcoholism should be classified as one disorder or two. *Alcoholism* appeared in the DSM-I as a sociopathic personality disturbance (imagine saying that at an Alcoholics Anonymous meeting: *Hi, I'm Sarah and I'm sociopathically disturbed*).[5] In the DSM-II, it was classified as a non-psychotic personality disorder. The DSM-III no longer used the term *alcoholism* and referred to it as *substance use disorder,* which was divided into two subtypes: *substance abuse* and *substance dependence.* What was the difference? Few could say. Some speculate that *abuse* referred to drinking problems that incurred negative social, legal, or occupational consequences, and *dependence* meant withdrawal, but the DSM-III wasn't clear.[6] The split remained in the DSM-III-R and the DSM IV. The DSM-5 combined abuse and dependence into the broadly defined and easy-to-be-diagnosed-with *substance-related and addictive disorders*.[7]

At the time, I only needed one of the following symptoms to qualify for a substance abuse disorder: a failure to fulfill major work obligations (not yet), interpersonal problems (check), drinking in dangerous situations (check), substance-related legal problems (not yet). A substance dependence disorder required only three of the following: tolerance (check); withdrawal (check); larger amounts taken over a longer period than intended (double check); persistent desire or unsuccessful efforts to stop (check); "a great deal of time" spent to get, use, or recover from alcohol (drinking was my job); activities no longer participated in (check); continued drinking despite knowing there's a problem (absolutely).[8] I would have aced the test.

Yes, I drank fast and plenty, and it hit me hard, but either no one noticed or they did but didn't care. Yes, I blacked out, but I didn't take nips of alcohol first thing in the morning. Yes, alcoholism ran in families and it ran in mine, but I wasn't an alcoholic and could stop anytime.

———

When I got home from work the night before my first day at the writing center, Chris was already asleep. He had to be up at 4 a.m. to make it to the bakery. Cappy brushed against my legs and let out a *mer-ow*. I brought my finger to my lips: "Shh." She let out another, louder *mer-ow*.

Not a drop. All I had to do was hang up my coat, put down my bag, go into the bathroom, turn on the light, and start getting ready for bed.

The rest seemed to come from someone else: the kitchen, a wineglass, the bottle of red on the counter. As I uncorked it, I paused, picturing myself in the writing center, a student asking me to look over his essay, my eyes scanning the page, hitting on commas and letters and periods, and not being able to tell him if it was correct. The rules. I didn't know the rules.

One glass turned into two . . . then three. As I drank, my thoughts looped: *the writing center . . . wines to order . . . sommelier study group . . . commas*. I went to the bookshelf. My legs felt heavy. I scanned the spines for a grammar book I knew was there but couldn't find.

Back at the table, I lifted my still-half-full glass to my lips. It was simple: pour it down the sink. I stood and went to the kitchen. Just one more sip . . . and another . . . and . . .

My lips drew tight. *Drunk. I was drunk.* It had happened before . . . many times . . . and had been happening more often. I tried to smile but couldn't. A kind of paralysis spread to my arms and legs. I pitched forward and leaned against the counter and . . .

The next morning, the alarm went off and I showered. Chris had long since been at work. I didn't remember changing and getting into bed. In the kitchen, my wineglass was washed and in the dish rack already dry. The bottle I'd finished was rinsed and in the recycling bin.

The bike ride down the hill was a rush. I was still drunk. Downtown, I locked up my bike to a rack and waited for the bus. The man next to me smelled of alcohol. No, I smelled of alcohol.

On the bus to North Seattle, I ate the bagel I'd made. It sopped up whatever alcohol—if any—was left in my stomach. Half an hour later, my head started to pound.

I made it to the writing center five minutes late. The other tutors were seated at the various tables listening attentively to the director. I slipped in and sat in the back. No one would notice. I'd covered the smell of alcohol by chewing peppermint gum and dabbing lavender oil on my wrists.

As the director spoke, an older woman with short, graying hair interrupted her twice. It would have been annoying except everything the woman said about the semester's assignments and how best to work with students was helpful.

The director finished and introduced the woman as Evelyn, who would be leading a professional-development mini lesson. Evelyn stood up and used a sandwich board to outline her main points: *nominative case, objective case, possessive case, case in opposition, nominative of address.*

I nodded at what she said but had no idea what she was talking about. Cases were way out of my league. Around me, the others nodded too. I wondered if theirs were truthful.

———

That afternoon at home, I went to the bookshelf and pulled out the grammar book. It felt heavy in my hands. I'd study. At the next meeting, I'd nod for real.

My wineglass was still on the dishrack. Seated at the table, I read: *case*, *number*, *person*. A dot flashed in the corner of my right eye. I went to the bathroom. My migraine pills weren't in the medicine cabinet. I searched my bag. Finding them, I popped one in my mouth and swallowed it with water. My migraines called for a dark room. I closed the blinds in the bedroom and lay on the bed.

The lightshow started. A firework display of white light started as a dot and grew—dot by dot—until my vision was impeded and I couldn't move. My hands started to tingle. Then my face. The flashing light grew larger. The pain started in the top right of my skull, a concentrated, leaden pain.

I thought, *Brain hemorrhage*. My breathing grew shallow and merged with a sharp pain in my chest. I wanted to call Chris, call an ambulance, but I couldn't see. So I lay there, monitoring the pain in my heart and the frequency of the flashes of light.

Cappy hopped onto the bed, startling me. She walked across my stomach, nuzzled in the crook of my neck, and purred.

I woke to the sound of Chris coming in the door. The aura was gone.

He sat on the edge of the bed and asked if I was okay. I said I'd had a migraine and clutched my chest. "I think something's wrong with my heart."

He smiled though not unkindly. "I think maybe you just had too much to drink last night."

———

An hour later, we sat on the blue plastic chairs of the emergency waiting room. I'd insisted on going. I was dying. I had to be dying.

The words *chest pain* should have gotten me in right away, but my blood pressure and oxygen levels and temperature must have told them that whatever was wrong with me, it wasn't urgent. My symptoms weren't severe enough to warrant immediate care.

An attendant called my name. We followed him and then a nurse to the triage area. I put on a hospital gown. Chris held both our coats in his arms. He leaned against the wall, his head back.

I sat on the gurney. The metal was cool against my leg. The thin white paper crumpled beneath me.

The doctor pulled back the curtain and said a confident hello. Chris said he'd wait outside and left, cradling both our coats. The doctor studied my intake forms. He shined a light into my eyes, looked inside my mouth, and peered inside each of my ears. I lay down. He pressed on my belly, asking if it hurt. I said no.

He told me to sit up. As he pressed the glands of my neck and pressed his stethoscope to my chest, I told him I'd had a migraine and my heart had felt as though it was being squeezed through a sieve. "It was like I was having a heart attack."

He raised his eyebrows and said that as a twenty-seven-year-old woman with no history of heart trouble in her family, I likely wasn't having a heart attack. "Are you experiencing more stress in your life?"

I said, "Not really." Although with my new job and Seattle not being what we'd hoped and feeling, well . . . hungover most of the time, I guess I was.

He picked up my forms and wrote something I couldn't see. "Because," he said, still writing, "stress can cause somatic symptoms."

Somatic symptoms. Psychosomatic. Psycho.

He slipped his pen into the pocket of his white coat.

They did an EKG. The doctor returned. Normal.

The pain, the same pain from that morning, pierced my heart. I asked if he thought we should do some more tests.

"You may want to consider talking to someone to help with any stress you may be feeling."

"What if it's not just stress?"

The doctor nodded curtly. "I'm pretty sure it's stress."

I dressed and went to Chris, kissed him, and told him what the doctor said. He shook his head, dismayed, as if to say, *See? Nothing's wrong with you.*

———

Malingerer—someone who purposely feigns or exaggerates illness for profit. The malingerer pretends to be sick to get out of work, military service, jury duty, a party. Or for disability, worker's comp, sympathy, care, attention. The malingerer is an opportunist who lies about the most important thing we have: our health.

But my heart pains were real. And the headaches. And the ringing in my ears. And the adrenaline rushes. And . . .

Hypochondriac, maybe. The hypochondriac produces bodily suffering where there is none. She either avoids doctors or compulsively seeks help from them, often getting second and third opinions, only to end up as unconvinced of her health as when she started. She's a burden, sapping the energies of family and friends, using up taxpayer money, and draining medical resources.[9]

Hypochondria was once treated as a physical illness but eventually was thought of as a mental disorder that manifests in physical symptoms. The word's very etymology is bodily. *Hypokhondria*—*hypo* meaning "under" and *khondria* meaning "cartilage"—refers to the soft part of the sternum between the ribs and the navel. Early physicians believed hypochondriacal symptoms were caused by a buildup of black bile in the stomach.[10] By the seventeenth century, hypochondria was considered the result of disordered thinking projected onto the body. During the eighteenth century, physicians classified it as a nervous reaction that resulted from privilege and weak nerves. It was most often diagnosed in wealthy, educated men.[11]

During the DSM era, hypochondria continued to be categorized as a psychosomatic illness. The DSM-I described *hypochondriacal neurosis* in Freudian terms as a neurotic condition that resulted from unconscious conflicts. The DSM-III referred to it as *hypochondriasis*.[12] The DSM-IV classified it under *somatoform* (body) *disorders*. The DSM-5 subsumed it under *somatic symptom* or *illness anxiety disorder*.

Today, hypochondria is considered long-term and debilitating.[13] The hypochondriac takes each pain as a sign of a deadly illness and rejects reassurance from health care professionals. She self-diagnoses with disease after disease. Her physical symptoms have no detectable cause.

If I'd seen a psychiatrist, I probably wouldn't have been diagnosed with hypochondriasis. It wasn't a popular DSM diagnosis at the time.[14] Possibly, that psychiatrist would have filed me under *generalized anxiety disorder* or a personality disorder or placed me on the obsessive-compulsive-disorder spectrum.[15]

If I'd seen a psychologist, she would have asked me to talk through the underlying trauma (I had none) or stress (I had relatively little) behind my hypochondria. If trained in cognitive behavioral therapy, she might have shown me how to break down my thoughts, question my assumptions, and recognize the way I jumped to conclusions, catastrophizing every ache and pain.

But I didn't see a psychiatrist or a psychologist; instead, I drank.

———

The night before my first day of tutoring I vowed not to drink. It went as well as you might expect: a glass of wine . . . and then another . . . and . . . When I arrived at the center, the director gave me another tour. She showed me the forms to fill out for each student.

Evelyn entered and sat at one of the tables. From her bag, she pulled her own reference books (the shelves were lined with many to choose from) and red pens, a glasses case, and a coffee thermos.

The director asked if I had any questions. I shook my head and sat at the table farthest from Evelyn. My stomach growled. It felt raw. My mind was so foggy that it seemed impossible to tutor anyone in anything.

I got up and gathered my own stack of reference books from the bookshelf. As I passed Evelyn's table, she slipped on a pair of horn-rimmed glasses and introduced herself. She was a retired writing and rhetoric professor and had been working at the center—for fun—since she'd retired.

The door to the center opened, and the first student walked in. My head started to pound. I sat at my table and tried to look busy. He headed toward Evelyn.

Before he sat down, Evelyn turned to me: "Would you . . . ?"

"Oh, no." I made it sound as if I were doing her a favor. "That's okay. You take him."

Evelyn took all three students who came in that morning. During my half-hour lunch break, I sat on a concrete bench and ate the egg salad sandwich I'd brought. The campus was crowded with students. The sandwich made my stomach feel better but did nothing to clear my head.

When I returned, Evelyn stood.

A sense of panic came over me. "Where are you . . . ?"

She smiled. "Lunch."

A student walked in. He beelined in my direction. That same pain pierced my heart.

He sat across from me and pulled out the paper he was working on. Evelyn passed our table.

Another pain—this time in my side. Deep. My liver? Pancreas? Spleen? Something was wrong . . . really wrong.

I asked the student's name. He told me. My stomach seized. I asked what he needed help with. He hesitated. I waited. He pulled out an assignment sheet and handed it to me: *Brainstorm on a topic for . . .* Relief flooded me. He needed to brainstorm an essay. That, I could do.

———

Alcoholism has most recently been accepted as a disease, particularly in recovery communities like AA, which tells its members it's chronic and that they're powerless over it. Despite this, AA cofounder Bill

Wilson didn't actually consider it a "disease entity" though he was willing to call it an illness.[16]

As far as the science goes, Wilson was right: It has no known biological cause. Many consider it to be a mix of personality (sociopathy),
genetics, socioeconomics, and (a very loaded assumption) ethnicity.[17]
People are as likely to recover through clinical intervention as without it.

The mind-neurosis/brain-disease dilemma has troubled psychiatry
since the late nineteenth century. Two major figures epitomized the
dichotomy: Emil Kraepelin and (of course) Freud. Kraepelin is often
referred to as the father of biological psychiatry (though at the time,
biological meant autopsying brain matter as neurotransmitters hadn't
yet been discovered), Freud the father of psychoanalysis. Kraepelin
investigated the brain; Freud theorized the mind. Kraepelin believed
mental illnesses were caused by external factors and biology; Freud
that they were triggered by childhood trauma, psychic conflict, and
sexual fantasies. Kraepelin tended those with serious mental illnesses
in asylums; Freud listened to the worried well in the city. Kraepelin focused on the course and prognosis of mental disorders; Freud hunted
for their hidden causes. Kraepelin classified; Freud generalized (often
based on reflections about himself and maybe one or two patients).

Psychiatric philosophy and practice has moved between these two
theories and approaches. During the late nineteenth century, the brain
was thought to hold the answers to what was referred to as insanity and
"idiocy." Psychiatrists, nearly all of whom treated the most severely ill
in asylums, were often more interested in conducting autopsies than
treating patients.[18] (The 1880 census defined seven types of mental illness: three divided the agitated-violent from the depressed-nonviolent;
the other four were paralysis, dementia, alcoholism, and epilepsy.)

Then psychiatry changed. During the first part of the twentieth
century, Freudian ideology and methods dominated clinical practice
and universities. Like Freud, many psychiatrists went to cities and
towns to treat the upper classes with mild complaints. (Freud was
something of a snob. He would only see patients of a certain education, class, and age, and refused to see psychotic patients, adolescents,

and anyone older than fifty on the grounds that they would not be properly receptive to psychoanalysis. The general population, he once wrote in a letter, was "trash.")[19] Psychoanalytic theories of the neurotic mind became the vogue, like those in Freud's 1901 treatise, *The Psychopathology of Everyday Life*, which turned simple acts like forgetting a name or saying the wrong word into evidence of unconscious desires and repressed memories.

Of the two manuals that predated the DSM, *The Statistical Manual for the Use of Institutions for the Insane* favored a biological explanation whereas the *War Department Technical Bulletin, Medical 203* relied primarily on a neurosis-based one. In 1918, the American Medico-Psychological Association (later renamed the American Psychiatric Association) compiled the *Statistical Manual* to obtain data about who received care in mental hospitals and asylums.[20] It was used by hospitals for record-keeping but not widely beyond that.[21] This was due, in part, to the fact that the powerful psycho-biologist Adolf Meyer, psychiatrist-in-chief at the Johns Hopkins School of Medicine, didn't approve. Meyer believed mental illnesses were caused by a combination of biology and "reactions" to life circumstances that presented as illnesses. (Chalk him up as one of psychiatry's many controversial figures. He was involved in the eugenics movement and supported a treatment that removed—one by one—the "infected" organs of people with schizophrenia.)[22] The *Statistical Manual* outlined twenty-one diagnoses: twenty applied to those with psychosis with an assumed biological basis and just one to those without psychosis (neurosis). It was the dominant classification system used until the early 1940s.

In 1946, a group of mental health professionals, under the auspices of the U.S. Army, published *Medical 203* to support servicemen and veterans experiencing trauma and psychological distress.[23] *Medical 203* focused on people who had experienced neurotic reactions to stressful life situations, not those who were hospitalized. Unlike the diagnoses in the *Statistical Manual*, most of the categories outlined in *Medical 203* were considered temporary and treatable. *Medical 203* was intended for the general public.

The DSM arose out of these two approaches and the tension be-tween the brain-disease and mind-neurosis theories. The DSMs I and II allied with the mind-neurosis side. The DSMs III, III-R, IV, IV-TR, and 5 moved to the brain-disease side, which is where we are now.

———

On a cloudy, drizzling morning, while Chris was at work, I opened the window. Cool, damp air came in. I sat on the couch to read *A Moveable Feast*. Cappy snuggled in my lap.

The pages of the book consoled me. Literally, the pages. Just hold-ing them. Even if just for half an hour. Not that book in particular; any book would have done.

In *A Moveable Feast*, Ernest Hemingway's posthumously published memoir (though he said it should be taken as fiction), he romanticizes his years in Paris during the interwar period as a member of what Ger-trude Stein called the Lost Generation. It would be another five years before I read all his novels and learned that his macho-celebrity public posturing and the systemic sexism and racism in the literary world had as much to do with his standing as "the great American writer" as his actual writing did.[24] It would be another ten years before I read Toni Morrison's critique of his racism in *To Have and Have Not* and *The Garden of Eden*.[25] But at the time, I knew little and didn't take issue with *A Moveable Feast*—not even the way Hemingway fawned over the antisemitic modernist poet Ezra Pound.[26]

Hemingway's memoir offers an account of an evening with F. Scott Fitzgerald at a bar in Paris. Unsympathetically, Hemingway describes Fitzgerald having a physical reaction to champagne. Fitzgerald starts to sweat. The skin on his face tightens and looks like "a death mask." No one had ever described that strange paralysis that came over me when I drank. It seemed so awful, so pathetic to think of Fitzgerald—and me—like that.

It would be years before I learned that Fitzgerald might have been suffering from alcohol poisoning, alcohol sensitivity, and/or chronic al-cohol exposure. Not everyone gets a dopamine hit or an endorphin rush when they drink;[27] some are prone[28] to anxiety, depression (alcohol is a depressant), stress, and other, more toxic effects.[29] In chronic alcohol exposure, the neural circuits are altered,[30] which leads to increased sensitivity, tolerance, and dependence. In extreme cases, not everyone vomits (a sign the body is desperately trying to expel the alcohol to save you); some experience hypothermia.[31] Because alcohol causes blood vessels under the skin to dilate and inhibits the body's ability to shiver, a person's body temperature can fall too quickly. If the person starts to sweat, as in Fitzgerald's case, the result can be an alcohol-induced coma or death.

I continued to read. Hemingway and Fitzgerald travel to Lyon together. Their day starts with whisky and moves through four bottles of wine by the afternoon. After getting caught in a rainstorm (they're driving a convertible Renault with no top), they decide to spend the night in a local hotel. The two men's clothes are soaked through. Fitzgerald worries about catching pneumonia. Hemingway taunts him by providing the details of the illness (fever and delirium). Hemingway tells him to drink more wine, saying it counteracts pneumonia (it doesn't). Fitzgerald insists he has a temperature. Hemingway feels his forehead and gruffly says he's fine and to have a whisky. Fitzgerald becomes more panicked about the illness he's certain he has. Hemingway responds by mocking him more.

It wasn't so much Hemingway's callousness in the scene that bothered me (taunting Fitzgerald with pneumonia's symptoms was akin to letting a hypochondriac loose on WebMD); it was his cruelty for including it. Fitzgerald didn't deserve to be portrayed as a pitiful hypochondriac who couldn't hold his drink.

———

The two conditions might be connected: hypochondria and alcoholism. The direction of the relationship is unclear. Does the hypochondriac self-medicate with alcohol or does alcohol use lead to hypochondria? Some hypochondriacs self-medicate with alcohol.[32] They use it to numb the extreme sensations in their bodies that make them believe they're ill and going to die. But repeated exposure to alcohol has been found to reduce the brain's ability to process fear, which may trigger hypochondria, an excessive reaction to bodily sensations.[33]

If someone had promised to free me of one condition if I agreed to adopt and label myself with the other—hypochondriac or alcoholic—I'd have chosen alcoholic. Alcoholism seemed to offer a way out: quit drinking. Problem solved. The only part that didn't appeal to me was having to live my whole life AA-style, introducing myself as an alcoholic and carrying around a coin though I no longer drank alcohol or met the DSM's criteria for alcohol dependence syndrome.

Hypochondria would have been worse. It wasn't just a string of irrational thoughts; it was a bedrock of beliefs, convictions that came without warning and stayed as long as they pleased. They were unshakable even in the emergency room, where it was so clear that nothing physical was wrong. I'd have to live as an obsessive, assuming every pain to be fatal and ignoring the doctors who told me otherwise. As a depressive, I'd diagnose myself again and again and either avoid doctors so I could believe in my symptoms or compulsively seek help from them in the hope that one would finally agree that I was ill.

My hypochondria started with a strange, dislocating sensation like someone had pulled me out of my body. Each sensation—a pain, an ache, a ringing, a twinge, a rush—confirmed that death was imminent: a migraine was a hemorrhage waiting to happen, a stomachache meant cancer, dizziness signaled a brain tumor. The thought *I'm going to die* would arrive and run on repeat.

Alcoholic, definitely . . . maybe . . .

———

The night before the Master Sommelier exam in Las Vegas, Chris and I went out for an expensive dinner and drank expensive wine. The next day—hungover—I sat in a hotel conference room with about fifty other people. The master sommelier stood at the front and guided us through tastings.

Normally, I would have enjoyed holding a glass of white wine up to the light to assess its color and clarity. I'd have swirled my glass along with everyone else, examining the wine's legs. It would have been a pleasure to raise the glass to my nose and smell butter and apple and so much oak as to be certain it was a California Chardonnay. But the room felt crowded and the lights overhead too bright. I felt foggy and sick, like something toxic was inside me.

At the end of the day, Chris met me and we walked the Strip. A middle-aged man came toward us, weeping. I wondered if he'd been gambling and how much money he'd lost.

Another dinner . . . more wine . . . the vague memory of the two of us riding a roller coaster late that night. The next day, I received my results. I passed. At a small ceremony, the master sommelier bestowed on me a basic certification pin and a diploma. I took home the course booklet as a keepsake.

A few weeks after the exam, while Chris was at work, I sat at our kitchen table typing on my laptop. I'd started writing poems. They were short and manageable and I could work on them in bursts.

I'd stopped drinking most days . . . sometimes . . . though not entirely . . . but never on the nights before I had to tutor. At the writing center one day, Evelyn explained the nominative case. (It's just an unfamiliar term for a noun used as the subject of a verb: *Sarah drinks alcohol* or *Sarah worries about her health.*) I watched and studied her, how she helped students, directing them to pay attention to the words on the page and how their order gave them meaning. When we worked the same shift, I tried to speak quietly to the student I was working with, so Evelyn wouldn't hear me mix up rules or give the wrong information. There were still so many gaps in my knowledge of punctuation, so many ways I was confused.

II

4

Un-joined

Billie Holiday's raw, throaty voice had been playing on the radio for hours. New York City's public radio station was devoting an entire day to her music. I sat on the kitchen floor of my Brooklyn studio apartment unwrapping my mugs and plates which had been bundled in newspaper for the move. My third move of the year. My second move alone.

Chris had been offered an acting job in New York. We'd rented a room in a Brooklyn loft we shared with five other people. The room was really a storage space with a mattress. He fell into a routine of rehearsals and seeing friends and waiting tables; I waited tables and drank.

I ended our relationship carelessly and harshly. Instead of dealing with my drinking and my hypochondriacal thoughts, I convinced myself I was in love with someone else. That man, it turned out, was married (though he'd forgotten to tell me) and already having an affair with someone else.

While I was living in a sublet, my drinking hit a crisis point. I don't remember a lot about the months that followed. Flashes come: bottles of wine, tears; nights at bars alone, thinking how great it was that my love for whisky had deepened.

One flash lasts too long: candles lit, the room blurry, and the thought that I wanted to die. The next morning, the thought felt thick, factual, confirmation of the images and thoughts I'd had in Chicago. By midmorning, once toast and eggs had seemed to sop up the whisky from the night before, the ideation seemed melodramatic, something out of a bad movie.

Eventually, I quit drinking—just like that. No tapering off. No AA meetings; not once did I think of myself as an alcoholic. No final drink. No morning that marks the start of my sober life. I'd had enough. The panicked thoughts of illness and dying went away, too. And I found a home, a garden apartment in Brooklyn.

On the radio came a live recording of Holiday singing "Stormy Weather." Her torchy voice was quiet at first: *Don't know why.* As a thirty-year-old white woman, I couldn't exactly lay claim to Holiday. With her performance of "Strange Fruit," a song about the lynchings of African Americans, she'd been embraced by the Civil Rights Movement. Still, she moved me more than any other singer. It wasn't just her voice with its layers and moods; it was the way she worked the lyrics. Her unexpected hesitations joined some words—*no sun-up in the sky*, *keeps-raining all the time*—and severed others—*my man and I ain't to-gether*, *stormy wea-ther*.

Outside, it was a hazy spring morning. I was weary and well. Normal weary. Grieving-the-loss-of-a-six-year-relationship weary. I'd never join my life to Chris's. The question as to whether I'd take his last name and drop my own or hyphenate the two would never come up.

I'd started running a few miles a day five days a week. It had nothing to do with losing weight. It was about pacing and my breath and fresh air and moving my body and letting thoughts pass through.

*Mer-ow*ing, Cappy strolled into the kitchen, her tail up in greeting. Even for a Siamese, she was talkative. She held long conversations with me and I with her. People with children and husbands and wives and partners and too-many-friends-to-keep-up-with don't have the same attachment to their pets as those who are more solitary. I was the giver of catnip, the supplier of special wet food and canned tuna, the purveyor of behind-the-ear and under-the-chin scratches and nose kisses and tummy rubs and brushings.

As I scratched between her ears, she started to purr. She lifted her chin to allow me to scratch there, too. When I released my hand, she rubbed against my back, slunk around, and nosed her way onto my lap.

Holiday's voice trailed off, supplanted by applause and shouts. The deejay introduced a recording of "Solitude." The song started with its misleading trill, which made it seem as if what was to come would be delightful. After less than a beat of silence, Holiday elided the first three words, so they sounded like one: *In-my-solitude.*

My leg had fallen asleep. I nudged Cappy and slid her off my lap. From the cupboard I pulled down a can of wet food. She *mer-ow*ed and rubbed against my legs as I spooned the wet food into her bowl.

After she'd eaten, I went to the fridge and pulled out the vial of insulin. I followed the vet's instructions, shaking the vial until the liquid turned milky white, cleaning the rubber stopper with rubbing alcohol, drawing air into the syringe to the number of units prescribed, injecting the air into the vial to keep the pressure stable, turning the bottle over, making sure the needle was immersed in the liquid, and drawing the correct amount of insulin.

It seemed like too much insulin. The vet had instructed me to increase the dose—and increase it again, and again. We'd gone through vials that once lasted us twelve weeks in three. When I told the vet Cappy didn't seem to be getting better, she reassured me it would be fine. Everything would be fine.

I put Cappy on the single bed that doubled as my couch and rubbed her back. She settled in. I pinched a fold of skin between her shoulder blades, lifted it, and inserted the needle. With my thumb, I pressed the plunger until the syringe was empty.

———

Grief is usually defined as the distress felt after a person's death, not a breakup. It's the loss of someone dear—a child, a parent, a spouse, a friend. It's immediate and profound. The stomach sinks. The chest hollows. The body feels empty.

Maybe I didn't feel grief. Maybe it was anguish, which is more punishing. Or woe, which is inconsolable. Or sorrow, which is imbued with guilt and remorse.

I didn't know because my emotions were mostly foreign to me. Except for the obvious ones—happy, sad, scared, angry—I couldn't name them. Anguish, woe, and sorrow could have risen up and introduced themselves, and I wouldn't have recognized them.

————

The next morning, I ran my regular route: through McGolrick Park, one lap around the McCarren Park track, to the edge of the Hasidic neighborhood, and back along the East River. My route took me past the Domino Sugar Factory, which gave off a sweet smell. The other buildings along Kent Street were filled with artists and writers and actors and anyone else who couldn't afford Manhattan rents.

I spent the rest of the morning writing with Cappy on my lap. Before leaving the apartment that afternoon, I injected her with her dose of insulin. She *mer-ow*ed and walked me to the door.

When I arrived at the community center in Carroll Gardens where I taught English as a second language, my boss was still at her desk, working late. She waved distractedly. A fierce woman with short, reddish curly hair, she'd dedicated most of her life to the center. Even as Carroll Gardens had gentrified, she wouldn't sell the property, determined to make sure those east of the neighborhood's expensive row houses and boutique shops had access to ESL and GED classes.

I put down my coat and bag and pulled *The ESL Teacher's Activity-a-Day* grammar guide from the bookshelf. The pages were frayed at the edges. The cover promised to teach my students punctuation and grammar in five-minute lessons. Punctuation was listed under Mechanics, as if punctuation was straightforward and not riddled with nuances and vagaries.

At the copier, I made too many handouts. We were working on sentence endings: periods, exclamation points, question marks. My lesson plan was so packed I could have taught for six hours instead of three. It seemed unreasonable to think that I could, on Tuesday and Thursday nights, for just three hours each night, teach my students everything about the English language. Not that I knew everything. So as not to risk a student asking me grammar or punctuation questions I couldn't answer, I stuck mainly to vocabulary and simple sentences.

The classroom was in the basement. The musty smell had become familiar, even comforting.

The students who'd arrived early sat in uncomfortable, beat-up school desks. They were from all over the world, making the class a veritable Tower of Babel of languages: Arabic, Spanish, Polish, Amharic, Portuguese. Most juggled two or three jobs to take care of their families. How they managed to remain engaged, let alone awake, through class I didn't know.

The night went smoothly. It was easy to teach such determined students. They were so grateful for the knowledge it was my job to impart to them.

When I got home, the apartment was too quiet. I called Cappy's name. Nothing. She usually greeted me.

Finally, Cappy trotted around the corner—tail up as if in exclamation. That night, as usual, she slept with me under the covers, nuzzled against my stomach.

I still waited tables, lunch typically, at Gramercy Tavern, where—despite my onetime, fifteen-minutes-of-fame sommelier status—I was qualified to be a backwaiter. The next afternoon, my shift at the restaurant was long. We were slammed. I left feeling battered.

It was almost four by the time I got home. Cappy didn't come to greet me. I called her name as I hung my coat on a hook in the hallway. There was no sound, no sign of her.

In the main room, she lay on the floor. Her back legs were limp. I rushed to her, calling her name. She moaned a deep, throaty, harrowing *mer-ow*. The way it lingered on the *ow* seemed to come from her soul.

When I lifted her in my arms, her head lolled back. She didn't meet my eyes. I called her name again, clutching her to my chest. She let out another dazed *mer-ow*.

———

The cab to the veterinary hospital took too long. As we drove, Cappy didn't *mer-ow* so much as moan. I begged the driver to hurry.

On the Queensboro Bridge, we hit bumper-to-bumper traffic. Inside the carrier, she was slumped. Her eyes were glazed over like she was falling away. We were becoming un-joined.

In the dimly lit hallway of the hospital, while Cappy was being seen by the vet, I stood and waited. The word *neglect* came to mind. How easily I'd sometimes let her catnip remain out of reach under the bed or not bent down to pet her on my way out the door or got annoyed when she threw up on my comforter—again.

The nurse called me into the examination room. The vet was a tall man with dark hair. His chin was dimpled.

Cappy lay on the exam table covered by a blanket. She looked less dazed. As I scratched between her ears, she started to purr.

"She's better," I said, my voice rising with hope.

He explained that it was the IV solution they'd given her.

"She's purring."

He told me that cats don't just purr when they're happy. They learn to purr when they're a few days old and do it to communicate with their mothers. They also do it when they're in distress. And when they're sick. Purring occurs when a cat inhales and exhales, moving the muscles in the vocal cords, causing air to vibrate as it's pushed through. The frequency of the vibration has been found to promote bone and muscle growth and mend fractures and wounds.[1] Sometimes, they purr when they're dying.

He suspected that cancer had prevented her from absorbing the insulin. Did I want to have her tested for cancer? I asked if I should. He paused a little too long. Most likely, he said, it was cancer. Or the insulin wasn't administered properly.

I looked away and down at the scuffed tile floor.

Either way, he said, the prognosis wasn't good. The other option was to euthanize her.

I asked if he thought euthanasia was cruel.

He said if he thought it was, he wouldn't be a vet.

I had a moment to decide—literally ten minutes. The vet and the nurse left the room. Cappy lay on the table, purring. She was the closest living being to me. I'd lived with her for over a decade.

The bureaucratic process of putting her to sleep entailed many forms. In the hall, the nurse had me sign one to show I'd chosen communal cremation, one attesting she hadn't scratched or bitten anyone in the past ten days, and one stating I authorized the procedure. Payment was expected up front.

When I returned to the examination room, a clump of fur was missing from Cappy's leg where they'd shaved for the injection of a sedative. I tried to look into her eyes, to bond with her one last time, but as the sedative took hold, she fell away again.

The vet filled the syringe with what he told me was the euthanasia solution. The color was a shockingly bright blue. It was an overdose amount of a barbiturate, he explained. After he injected it, it would put her in a deep sleep, stop her breathing, and send her into cardiac arrest, which, supposedly, she wouldn't feel.

As he made the injection, I turned away. Minutes passed. Then the vet said she was "gone."

He and the nurse left the room. Cappy lay on her side, her mouth slightly open, her tongue protruding. Her eyes weren't closed. I stayed with her—and cried—for the fifteen minutes they allowed me.

Too soon, the nurse came in and politely told me that my time was up. Communal cremation meant I didn't receive her ashes. Holding her empty carrier, I exited the sterile, wall-tiled building onto Seventy-Third Street.

As I walked and turned onto York, each step made me feel less there. The sun had set. The streetlights were on. A man carrying a briefcase passed me. I stopped, resisting the urge to ask if he could see me and if I was real.

———

The Swiss-American psychiatrist Elisabeth Kübler-Ross wrote that there are five stages of grief: denial, anger, bargaining, depression, and acceptance. Denial is marked by shock and confusion; anger by frustration and hostility; bargaining by reaching out to others; depression by helplessness and listlessness; acceptance by recognizing reality without struggling against it. Contrary to popular belief, she meant that these stages are experienced by the dying, not the bereaved. Kübler-Ross never intended them to be strictly interpreted because they aren't backed by scientific evidence.[2]

I felt hollow and empty. Maybe it was loss as defined by the *Oxford English Dictionary*: "the condition or fact of being lost, destroyed, or ruined; being deprived of or the failure to keep." Someone once told me I'd understand loss when Cappy died. I didn't understand it, but I experienced its trickery—how I could trip over something and think it was her or return from work and expect her to greet me. Some part of me believed we were still joined.

My reaction to her death was extreme: crying spells, trouble sleeping, discontentment with my work and writing. It was indulgent and privileged, I knew. How many people have the luxury to grieve a cat?

A lot, actually, but without Google, I couldn't type *grief* and *cat* into the computer and come up with forty-three million results.[3] Without access to Cornell University's College of Veterinary Medicine web page "Grieving the Loss of Your Cat," I couldn't learn that the Greek root of the word *euthanasia* means "good death" and reassure myself that maybe it wasn't necessary to feel weighed down with guilt. I couldn't find relief in a *Telegraph* article titled "My Cat Died, and It Affected Me as Much as Losing My Dad" and stop telling myself it was ridiculous to have such an outsize response to the death of a pet.

———

I started running every day—long distances. My regular route now stretched from my apartment in Greenpoint, up Bedford Avenue, over the Williamsburg Bridge, along the East River to Fourteenth Street, and back. My weekend route covered twelve miles and included a loop around Central Park. The run I called "the four bridges" was much longer: through Queens, over the Queensboro Bridge, down Manhattan, over the Brooklyn Bridge, through Dumbo, over the Manhattan Bridge, up the East River, over the Williamsburg Bridge, home. For months, I didn't take a day off.

After one of my runs, my left hip started to hurt. The pain was sharp but not so strong I couldn't ignore it and hope it would go away. Within a month, the pain was almost constant, lessening only when a deeper, numbing pain took hold. Still, every morning at six, I laced my running shoes and went too far, pushing too hard. I ran until the hollow emptiness was replaced by a temporary endorphin rush.

When blisters formed on my feet, I ignored them, too. It didn't seem to matter that I had trouble walking. Soon, I was hobbling to the subway and to work and to the grocery store.

But I could still run. A block or two of limping and I could lean forward and pitch my way into a jog. Eventually, the adrenaline kicked in and it was like the pain never existed.

———

If it had been 2020, a therapist or the internet or a women's magazine might have diagnosed me with anorexia athletica.[4] The term doesn't quite make sense: the word *anorexia* means a refusal to eat and those with anorexia athletica don't necessarily refuse food; they just exercise too much. They can become dependent on the endorphin rush (exercise addiction) or feel compelled to do it even though they don't enjoy it (exercise compulsion).

On the Compulsive Exercise Test (CET), I would have qualified.[5] If I couldn't exercise, I felt depressed, agitated, angry, irritable, frustrated, and anxious. After I exercised, I felt less stressed and tense, happier and more positive. (Wasn't that the point?) I exercised despite injury or illness because, I told myself, I was never too ill or injured.

If I'd accepted the diagnosis, I probably would have identified as "an anorexic" again. It would have made sense, given that I'd already been one and my mind was in a loop and my body was falling apart.

Exercise obsession isn't in the DSM, but a psychiatrist could have put me in the "Not Otherwise Specified" category in the DSM-IV or the "Other Specified Feeding or Eating Disorders" category in the DSM-5. "Not Otherwise Specified" (NOS) and its DSM-5 doppel-gänger "Not Elsewhere Classified" (NEC) are ways to diagnose where there is no diagnosis. They're used for those who don't meet the criteria of a diagnosis but *kind of* seem like they may have something *kind of* wrong with them in a way that *kind of* seems clinically significant (like it's affecting their daily lives and relationships). It's as if the DSM is saying, *Who cares if someone doesn't actually merit a diagnosis? Go ahead and level one anyway.*

———

A two-inch-long blister had spread across the arch of my foot. The pain would have been excruciating except that it was still puffy and hadn't yet burst. It was just there, bulbous and threatening.

I hobbled out of my apartment and down the block. My hip still throbbed. Gaining momentum, I launched into a jog. It would be a short run. A quick mile.

Five miles into it, my sock felt damp. I stopped and took off my shoe. The blister had popped. A clear pus soaked my sock. I put my shoe back on and ran home.

In my apartment, as if nothing had happened, I turned on the ste-reo and put on Billie Holiday's "There Is No Greater Love." In the Decca Records recording, Holiday's voice is smooth and confident. She doesn't hyphenate the lyrics, except two words: *greater-love.*

The blister didn't sting in the shower so much as singe. The pain distracted me from the guilt I'd been feeling for weeks. The guilt was the worst part: betraying Chris, putting Cappy to sleep.

I got out of the shower, toweled off, and dressed. Blood quickly seeped through my sock. The least I could have done was put on a Band-Aid or wear two pairs of socks. Or tape my foot. Or try Vaseline. I did none of these—no antiseptic, no bandage.

A friend I hadn't seen since long before Cappy died got in touch and we met for dinner. Afterward, as we walked down Second Avenue, she noticed I was limping. It was then that I felt the pain, as if only her words had made it real. Saying I was fine, I tried to keep walking but couldn't. I leaned against a building and pulled off my boot and sock. The blister—now a wound—was leaking blood and pus.

"Jesus," she said. "What's that from?"

I didn't see the harm in answering: "Running, I guess."

The look on her face was a mix of disgust and concern. "You should see my therapist."

"No," I said, putting on my boot, "it's okay. I'm fine."

———

A week later, my friend called and insisted. I agreed because I hadn't been able to run for two days. The guilt and the sinking feeling and the hollowness and the emptiness felt like they were about to swallow me.

By the time I reached the psychologist's office on Eighty-Fourth Street, not far from the veterinary hospital where Cappy had died, the sinking-hollow-emptiness increased. If I could just go for a run . . .

Her office was on the garden level. I rang the bell and was buzzed in. No one greeted me. No one was in the waiting room. It was dimly lit with dark-green carpeting, antique furniture, and faded floral-print curtains. I sat in a large armchair and sifted through issues of *People* magazine.

Five minutes passed. Then ten. I wondered if I had the wrong afternoon.

Finally, the psychologist came out. Slight of frame and probably in her sixties, she didn't apologize for being late.

The narrow windows in her office looked out onto Eighty-Fourth Street. Framed posters of abstract art hung on the walls.

She sat in a Victorian parlor chair at one end of a long, dark-wood coffee table. I sat in a similar chair at the other. Pen poised over the legal pad on her lap, she asked about my experiences with therapy. I told her I'd been diagnosed with anorexia at twelve and had seen a therapist.

She pressed me for details.

I told her.

She asked if I was eating.

"Yes."

She nodded disbelievingly and wrote something on her legal pad. We covered my family and childhood. Every word seemed weighty and consequential, as if she knew a truth I couldn't know myself.

I told her about Cappy and the vet and the hospital and while trying not to cry, started to cry. She didn't offer me a tissue, maybe because there was a box right there on the table between us and she expected me to get one myself. When she asked me if I had trouble sleeping or had lost interest in my work or hobbies, I said, "Maybe. Yes."

When our time was up, she sighed. Then she told me I had major depressive disorder. I still didn't know much about depression or any diagnosis. Depression was a well-worn topic in memoirs—Elizabeth Wurtzel's *Prozac Nation*, Lauren Slater's *Prozac Diary*, Andrew Solomon's *The Noonday Demon*—though I hadn't read any of them. It was, I thought, caused by a chemical imbalance. The diagnosis seemed self-explanatory: I had depression and it was major.

She went to her desk and wrote something on a pad. I should be on an antidepressant, she said, as if it was obvious.

The part of me that wanted to argue gave way to the part that thought the diagnosis could make sense. I'd been anorexic. And what about the images I'd had in Chicago? And my drinking? She was a licensed psychologist. In her expert opinion, I had a mental illness and clearly needed medication. I hadn't even told her about the suicidal thoughts or my blistered feet.

She handed me a piece of paper with the name and number of a psychiatrist. "He's great," she said.

As I stepped out onto Eighty-Fourth Street, the sinking-hollow-emptiness swelled in me. *Mental illness*. It felt so definitive, so final. I limped toward the subway, folding the paper with the psychiatrist's name and number in half and then into quarters and then into eighths and slipping it into my pocket.

As an emotion, depression has been written about for over two thousand years. Evidence of it can be found in writings from ancient Egypt and in medical textbooks from ancient Greece. Its characteristics haven't always been seen as problematic. Lethargy is a normal part of being human. So are despair, emptiness, negativity, and a lack of pleasure and interest in activities. Even social detachment is a common response to many situations.

As a diagnosis, depression dates back to the nineteenth century. Melancholia, as it was called, was rare and considered a serious illness.[6] *Fatigue* wouldn't get you a diagnosis, neither would *loss of interest or pleasure* or the ubiquitous *low mood*; only agitation, hallucinations, paranoia, and dementia would.

The DSM-III broadened the definition of depression and made it easy to diagnose.[7] All depression—mild or severe, neurotic or psychotic—was the same. By the end of the twentieth century, depression replaced anxiety as the most commonly diagnosed mental illness because approaches to the diagnosis changed.[8] Depression's "rise" was due in part to marketing by pharmaceutical companies that manufactured antidepressants but primarily because the DSM-III didn't distinguish between the symptoms of serious (melancholic) depression and mild (neurotic) depression.[9] The cause of a person's depression was also of little interest. For thousands of years, physicians had considered possible external causes, but with the DSM-III, the distinction between exogenous depression (caused by events, triggers, and stressors) and endogenous depression (caused, perhaps, by biology or genetics and treatment resistant) didn't factor in.[10] Major depressive disorder (MDD) changed little in the DSM-III-R, the DSM-IV, and the DSM-5 (although the DSM-5 got rid of the bereavement clause—more on that later). The result, as Allen Frances said, has been the "transformation of expectable sadness into clinical depression," as well as overdiagnosis and misdiagnosis: "If we try to diagnose everyone who really has major depression, inevitably we will misdiagnose many people who are simply having a rough patch in their lives that needs no medical label and requires no treatment."[11]

Did I require a label? Treatment? Did I even have "depression"?

———

On the evening of my birthday, I arrived at the community center to teach my ESL class. My boss was there working late on a grant that wouldn't give the center the amount of money it needed. At the copier, I made handouts describing the difference between *may* and *might*—*may* being stronger and showing more emphasis and *might* indicating a moment in the future: *She might feel better. She may feel better.*

I went over my lesson plan. The phone rang. My boss picked it up. I wanted to tell her about the sinking-hollow-emptiness and how scared I was it would never go away. The piece of paper with the psychiatrist's number sat on my kitchen table at home.

As I made my way down the stairs, louder voices than usual came from the classroom. On the landing, I heard, "Shh." The lights in the classroom went off. I walked in. The lights came on to scattered shouts of "Surprise!" A large, white-icinged cake sat on one of the desks. Blue balloons floated above the chairs. The students sang "Happy Birthday." They were so full of joy, so genuine that a mix of appreciation, endearment, and embarrassment flooded me. Though I knew little about them, I was more connected to them than anyone else in my life.

We ate the cake and "practiced conversation," meaning we talked and communicated as best we could. We played *Your House Is on Fire*, a game they loved. I divided them into pairs. In the game (it's a real game), Student A's house is on fire but luckily Student B is outside the house and calls to warn Student A. Student B happens to have a key to the house. The fire, it seems, isn't so bad that Student B can't risk her life to go inside and save whatever possessions Student A wants her to. Student A has to describe the objects Student B should rescue and where the objects are in the house. After they've described three objects, they switch roles.

That night, I may have taught them about the hyphen. We use the hyphen to link letters and words. It's all about connection. It unifies. It makes two one.

A seemingly simple punctuation mark, it's anything but. The rules are murky at best: Use it for compound adjectives, never with adverbs (*biologically caused mental illnesses*), and only when it might create confusion or unless a word looks odd without it (*pre-death, post-death*). The rules are always changing: *cry-baby* became *crybaby*, *death-bed* became *deathbed*. A hyphenated word can become one word or be eternally severed.

The hyphen's first known appearance was in treatises by the grammarian Dionysius Thrax in the second century BCE. Initially written at the bottom of the line (the sublinear hyphen), it bowed slightly. The Alexandrians must have loved it, given the way it clarified meaning at a time when no spaces separated words. The Greeks kept it up, giving it the name *hyphen* (which means "under one"). Its usage became common practice with the advent of Gutenberg's printing press, particularly the "marginal hyphen," which showed that a word had been broken over two lines of text.

After the students were gone, I went upstairs to the center's kitchen and washed the knife we'd used to cut the cake. The sinking-hollow-emptiness returned. *No. No. Not again.*

I pulled my phone from my bag and called Chris. We hadn't spoken in months. He didn't answer. I left a message asking him to meet.

A few days later, we sat at one of the cafés on Bedford Avenue. He drank a cappuccino. I had tea. His cheeks were flushed and his eyes bright. He told me about the record label he'd started and the show he was in. I didn't mention the psychologist or the MDD diagnosis or the running. (I'd tried not to limp on my way into the café.) But I told him a bit about the sinking-hollow-emptiness.

Sharply, he said, "You need to figure out what makes you happy."

Happy? Happy wasn't even on the table; all I wanted was for the sinking-hollow-emptiness to be gone.

When I got home, I unfolded the slip of paper with the psychiatrist's name and number and held it. Maybe I was sick. Maybe I did have major depression, clinical depression. I stood there, staring at the thin paper in my hand.

One factor might have saved me from an MDD diagnosis: grief. The DSM's early bereavement exclusion said that someone grieving could exhibit symptoms of depression without having MDD. It even stated as much: "a full depressive syndrome frequently is a normal reaction" to bereavement.[12] But allowing for grief would make MDD more difficult to diagnose. So the DSM-III-R stated that if grief lasted more than two months, a clinician might decide that "uncomplicated bereavement" had become MDD despite no changes in symptoms. Poof. Just like that. The DSM-IV further limited the bereavement clause. People, it seems, are only allowed to mourn the deaths of others, not the losses of jobs they've held for twenty years or houses that have burned down. The DSM-5 eliminated it altogether. Why? Because, as Allan Horwitz and Jerome Wakefield point out, the bereavement clause was "a compelling, clear, and major violation of [MDD's] validity."[13]

These were the DSM-IV years, and I wouldn't have qualified anyway. I was mourning a breakup and not Chris's death, and the death of a cat, not a person, and it had lasted almost half a year.

It must have been fairly easy for the psychologist to diagnose me— or anyone else—with MDD. According to the DSM-IV, I needed just five of nine symptoms to last over two weeks: low mood (sure), loss of pleasure and interest in most activities (check), significant change in appetite (yes), sleep disruptions (isn't that the nature of sleep?), slowness of physical and emotional reactions (perhaps), indecisiveness (maybe), inappropriate guilt (depends on your views on euthanasia). I could rule out fatigue or loss of energy and incessant thoughts of death or suicide or a suicide attempt.

In some ways, the DSM-IV tried to make it more difficult to be diagnosed with MDD. It specified that symptoms must be marked or "significant" and occur for at least two weeks. (Just two weeks?) It tried to create a "clinical significance" benchmark that required a person to exhibit "significant distress or impairment in social, occupational, or other important areas of functioning."[14] But it didn't define what "marked" or "significant" means.

The MDD criteria were so loose that depression had already become a false epidemic. As Allen Frances writes, a false epidemic occurs when three forces collide: DSM diagnostic criteria are loosened or altered; drug companies see a way to profit; and the media sensationalizes a disorder, christening it an "epidemic"—e.g., the "autism epidemic" or the "ADHD epidemic" or the "bipolar epidemic." As a result, people start to see the diagnosis in themselves and in their loved ones. They self-label and label each other, even seek it out.[15] No wonder that psychologist diagnosed me with such conviction.

———

The next morning, I put on my running shoes, grabbed my iPod, and went outside. After hobbling the first block, I broke into a jog, ignoring the pain. On my iPod came Billie Holiday singing "I Cover the Waterfront," recorded live in Cologne in 1954, five years before she died of cirrhosis of the liver. It was one of Holiday's signature songs. It's complex and haunting when Holiday sings it. In the Cologne recording, the lyrics often string together, giving them a deeper sense of loss: *I'm-standing-alone, des-olate-docks, my-heart, as-heavy-as-stone, in-search-of, my-love.* And the most telling line: *Will-the-dawn coming-on make-it-light?*

As my feet pounded against the tarred bike path over the Williamsburg Bridge, I heard a distant moan. A *mer-ow*. I turned down the volume on my iPod. A cat in pain. Not quite Cappy's signature, hyphenated *mer-ow* but close. I stopped and looked behind a dumpster where the sound seemed to be coming from. Nothing.

Along the East River came another *mer-ow*. At Fourteenth Street, another. On South Fourth Street, another.

None was real. One *mer-ow* had been a foghorn sounding from the

East River, another the hinges of a car door closing. A kind of halluci-
nation? Another reason to see the psychiatrist?

But something about the imagined *mer-ow*s comforted me. I
slowed my pace. When my hip started to throb, I picked up speed and
kept going, one step and then the next.

5

Ask Your Doctor

The classroom smelled of bleach, baby wipes, and pencil shavings. And apple juice. And pretzels. The shelves weren't lined with algebra textbooks; they held finger paint and crayons, plastic baggies, hand sanitizer, and boxes of surgical gloves.

Ms. Madelyn stood at the blackboard writing. We were waiting for the other six students, who were with the nurse. Only Natale and Kimberly—both sixteen, the only two girls, and the only two students in the room—sat at their desks. Natale had shoulder-length brown hair, the ends jagged. Her arms were crossed in front of her chest. Kimberly was doe-eyed.

I went through the handouts I'd brought. The arts organization I worked for sent writers into the New York City public schools to teach creative writing. (Calling me a professional writer was a stretch, but I'd been published and received fellowships to elite artist colonies and interviewed the poet Jack Gilbert for *The Paris Review* and so could be said to hover around the nether regions of "the literary world." I'd also enrolled in an MFA program in creative writing.) The arts organization had an impressive roster of authors who'd done what I was doing: June Jordan, Kenneth Koch, Phillip Lopate, Grace Paley, Muriel Rukeyser, Anne Sexton. For ten or twenty days, I was assigned to a school. I'd taught first graders in Queens to write haiku poems, seventh graders in the Bronx to write autobiographies, and tenth graders in Brooklyn to write short stories. More often than not, I taught special education students with severe mental and physical disabilities.

This high school in Queens was the kind a visiting writer wanted to be invited back to. I'd been there four years in a row. The bulletin boards hadn't been ripped down. The clocks worked. The teachers weren't burned-out, at least not in the special-education wing of the school.

Mr. Sam, the paraprofessional (an assistant teacher trained to work with children and teenagers with special needs), entered with the rest of the students in tow. All eight students in class had been diagnosed with autism severe enough for them to require an exclusive classroom.

Steadman and Xavier each wore a backpack slung over his shoulder. The backpacks were a trend, something Xavier started to be like the students in the regular-education part of the high school. Xavier's backpack was half-zipped and relatively empty, almost floating on his shoulder from the absence of books.

Kemal strode in. His school ID dangled from a lanyard around his neck. He put down his backpack next to his desk and headed in my direction.

When he reached me, he puffed out his chest. I knew what was coming.

He came close to me until his face was just a few inches from mine. "You talkin' ta *me*?" he asked in a Brooklyn accent fairly reminiscent of Robert De Niro's character, Travis Bickle, in *Taxi Driver*. "You talkin' ta me?"

This was his way of saying hello. The first time he did it, I bristled, jerking back as if he'd accosted me. But with each occasion, I felt less threatened. He was just acting out the movie the way teenagers do; it just happened to be a particularly violent movie.

"You talkin' ta me?"

I stepped back. "Okay, Kemal. Time to sit."

He nodded and went to his desk.

The twins, Bernard and Charles, entered with their nurse, Maria.

Their conditions were severe enough to warrant individualized care. Neither wore a backpack. One of the few ways I could tell them apart was that Charles yawned prodigiously and Bernard didn't. They sat at their desks and began flapping their hands. Called "stimming," this was a form of stimulation. Until Ms. Madelyn taught me about autism, I thought Bernard and Charles and the others displayed "autistic behaviors," but they were acting in accordance with their experience of the world. It was perfectly normal. Ms. Madelyn told me to treat them like any other students.

Reuben lumbered in, walking stiffly. He, too, had a backpack balancing light on his shoulder. As he passed, he said hello, his affect flat, his gaze down at the floor. He asked how I was. I told him I was fine and asked how he was. He said he was fine, too.

The students eventually settled down. I started to tell them the Greek myth of Icarus. The idea was that after reading (or listening to) a particular genre of writing (a myth, a poem, a short story), they would imitate it by writing their own. In special-education classes, most of the students—particularly those who were nonverbal—couldn't write. They either drew pictures or we prompted them with questions and wrote for them.

That day's assignment was to draw pictures of their own gods. Ms. Madelyn, Mr. Sam, Maria, and I moved around the room, checking the students' work, helping one student and then the next. Steadman was one of the few who could write. I peered over his shoulder at his paper. He'd written his name at the top of the page: *Steadman Kennedy Onassis.* That wasn't his name, but like many teenagers, he was obsessed with celebrities; his preoccupation happened to be with the Kennedys.

Noel, a nonverbal student, was drawing on his own. He could write, too. I stood behind him. On his paper were circles and ovals and squiggly lines. The figure he'd drawn resembled a gryphon—half lion, half eagle.

I sat with him. "Can I see?" I asked, almost reaching out to take his paper.

He raised one hand to his ear and the other to his mouth, a sign that he was becoming agitated.

I pulled back. Unlike Kemal, Noel had clearly defined boundaries when it came to personal space. "I'm sorry." I stood. "Good job."

As I went to work with Steadman, an unsettling edginess seemed to take hold of me. It had nothing to do with Noel. This wasn't the sinking-hollow-emptiness. My grief had subsided though it had taken almost two years. (I never called that psychiatrist and didn't see the psychologist again.) This was different—like being brittle and closed in at the same time.

On my way out of the school at the end of the day, I saw Jackie, one of the assistant principals. She had spiked, copper-colored hair. With ruddy exuberance, she asked me how it went. I said it went well. She smiled. "We're so, so, so happy to have you."

———

It was the height of the "autism epidemic." The U.S. Department of Education had reported a 657 percent rise in the national rate since 1993.[1] Autism supposedly affected 1 in 166 children. (That number would be said to grow to an implausible 1 in 54 by 2016.)[2]

When Leo Kanner at Johns Hopkins University identified autism in 1943, just one child in thousands were thought to suffer from it.[3] The term *autism* was borrowed from the Swiss psychiatrist Eugen Bleuler, who used it to describe a symptom of schizophrenia: predominance of the inner life and disassociation from the external world. Kanner defined autism as a developmental deficiency in sociability, communication, and activity marked by "altogether different" relations to other people and speech impairment.[4] The children he observed were characterized by self-isolation, repetition, and an obsession with sameness.

The American "epidemic" was helped along by media outlets and parents and teachers and social workers and psychologists and psychiatrists, but it was created by the DSM. Before autism appeared in the DSM, it was a rare disorder primarily associated with language and speech impairment. The DSM-III introduced autism as a standalone diagnosis from schizophrenia, characterized by impairments in communication, sociability, and responses to the environment. The DSM-III-R created an autism diagnosis centered on social functioning.[5] In addition, the criteria was substantially broadened, and a child or infant could be diagnosed at any age.

Parents, teachers, social workers, psychologists, and psychiatrists believed autism was a biological disease. Many studies supposedly showed its biological origins.[6] Genes were credited though no biological markers or causes had been found. Environmental factors were discussed, too. Pesticides and television were blamed.[7] Vaccines were incorrectly faulted. (*The Lancet*, which published the famous vaccines-are-to-blame article, retracted it after it was proven to be fabricated.)[8]

The DSM-IV so broadened the diagnostic criteria with the addition of Asperger's syndrome that the "epidemic" began in earnest. The Viennese pediatrician and eugenicist Hans Asperger coined the term Asperger's in 1944 to describe children with "autistic personality disorder."[9] He later wrote that this disorder was nothing like Kanner's "near psychotic" autism; Asperger's cases were "very intelligent children with extraordinary originality of thought and spontaneity of activity though their actions are not always the right response to the prevailing situation." The label Asperger's wasn't widely used to diagnose children until it appeared in the DSM-IV. Some on the task force that pushed to have it included later regretted it, saying there wasn't data to back up the second diagnosis.[10]

With so many children being diagnosed with Asperger's, parents started internet support groups and increased public awareness. Asperger's had cachet. Journalist Steve Silberman's 2001 article "The Geek Syndrome," published in *WIRED* magazine, connected Asperger's to the (highly lucrative) dot-com boom.[11] According to Silberman, Asperger's was a collection of "geek traits" originating in Silicon Valley, birthed by successful math-and-tech-obsessed parents.

The students in Ms. Madelyn's class didn't have Asperger's; they had straight-up Kanner autism. They were either "nonverbal" or used autistic speech patterns like echolalia (when I'd say hello to Kemal, he often repeated, "Hi, Kemal") or spoke of themselves in the third person ("Kemal wants a snack"). They suffered from intellectual disabilities and difficulty moving and walking. They didn't create relationships with others the way we think of relationships. During that time, they were the best part of my life.

———

A few weeks later, I was at the school again. The edginess had kept me up the night before; I'd paced my apartment. My thoughts spun, sharpening the edginess.

On my way to Ms. Madelyn's classroom, it grew stronger. I entered the room. The students said hello. They were calm. It was cloudy. I had no scientific evidence to support my belief that an overcast sky seemed to settle them. Maybe the sun was too stimulating.

We read "Ode to Broken Things" by the Chilean poet Pablo Neruda. Neruda wrote many odes in praise of people and things. Most were meditations on the ordinary: socks, the dictionary, a tuna for sale in the market.

Poetry was everything to me then—partly because I was in an MFA program in poetry and partly because poems could be read in stints, even when the edginess had crescendoed to a pitch. I read almost nothing else. No novels. Few essays. Never the news. When I felt well enough, I went to poetry readings at the 92nd Street Y, Poets House, the Bowery Poetry Club, or KGB Bar.

I stood at the front of the classroom and read Neruda's poem to the students:

Things get broken
at home
like they were pushed
by an invisible, deliberate smasher . . .

Life goes on grinding up
glass, wearing out clothes,

making fragments,
breaking down
forms,
and what lasts through time
is like an island on a ship in the sea,
perishable
surrounded by dangerous fragility
by merciless waters and threats.[12]

I read the last lines: "So many useless things / which nobody broke / but which got broken anyway."

The students seemed not to have heard me. Reuben stared at his paper and hummed. The twins sat with their backs to each other. Kemal rocked back and forth, a movement that some people with autism find soothing.

I reviewed the poem and asked what was broken. After I repeated the question a few times and gave examples, Bernard's hand shot up in the air. "The plates broke."

"And the house," Charles said.

They had been paying attention.

We started the writing exercise. Ms. Madelyn went to Steadman, Mr. Sam to Noel. Maria assisted the twins.

When I sat beside Natale, I asked what kinds of things break.

"Hearts," she said.

I wrote *Hearts break* on a sheet of paper.

"What else?" I asked, the edginess starting to return. "Do glasses break?"

"Hearts," she said again.

Her voice was barely audible, not just because she spoke softly but because my heart had started to pound. The sound echoed in my ears and through my mind, making it hard to hear her at all. It didn't pound in the way we normally think of it. It sounded and felt almost violent, as if it was trying to detach and break through my rib cage.

My bike ride home was five miles. I turned onto the most dangerous stretch—Vernon Boulevard. No bike lane. A truck barreled past, billowing exhaust. Sweat beaded down my face. It was June but not that hot. A car came so close to me that its side mirrors nearly swiped my handlebars.

The edginess didn't go away—not after I brought my bike inside my apartment, my legs so shaky I thought my knees were going to buckle. Not after I'd eaten what little dinner I could. Not as I lay in bed inhaling shallow sips of breath. Not as thoughts bombarded me, particularly the fear that I was losing my mind.

The rush of energy in my chest and pressure on my stomach stayed with me for days, becoming even more tormenting. All I wanted was for it to go away, which made it worse. It was like being rattled from the inside until I felt like I was splintering.

———

The human tendency toward anxiety goes back thousands of years. In ancient Greece and Rome, Epicurean and Stoic philosophers offered tips on how to avoid it.[13] (Spoiler: Stop worrying about the past and fearing the future.) In seventeenth- and eighteenth-century medical textbooks, along with the first descriptions of panic attacks, it was listed as part of melancholia. The symptoms were severe: hallucinations, mania, and delirium. In the nineteenth and early twentieth centuries, Kraepelin saw it not as a disorder but a symptom of many disorders, including manic-depression; to Freud, it was its own neurosis.

Anxiety was classified and reclassified with each edition of the DSM. In the DSM-I, it was listed as the main characteristic of psychoneurotic disorders and was used almost synonymously with neurosis. (The 1950s and 1960s are often referred to as "the Age of Anxiety," to use W. H. Auden's phrase, but it wasn't the anxiety we know today. Its symptoms were more typical of depression: sadness, malaise, headaches, fatigue, loss of appetite.) The DSM-III moved away from promoting anxiety as a neurosis and broke it into nine separate conditions, including phobias, panic disorder, generalized anxiety disorder, obsessive-compulsive disorder, and post-traumatic stress disorder

(PTSD). The DSM-IV added acute stress disorder as an anxiety sub-type. The DSM-5 placed anxiety on a series of spectra with OCD and trauma- and stressor-related disorders.

It seems so mild: *anxiety*. Worry, nervousness, unease. But the mere presence of it has been shown to increase the chances of suicidal ideation and suicide.[14] Anxiety makes a person feel besieged and threatened when there's no threat. Those rushes of energy I felt, the shakiness and edginess and splintering and catastrophic thoughts made me ten times more likely to end up in the dark place I eventually did.

———

I just needed "to relax." In yoga classes, I stood at the top of my mat and *om*ed and breathed and stretched and "twisted the tension from my body" as the teacher said. Someone told me to rub the mastoid bone behind my ears, which I did every morning and every night. I bought Chinese herbs at a store in the East Village—the root of some plant I can't remember. It looked like blackened tree bark and smelled like a rotting dog. (I know that smell: A stray dog died in the empty lot next to the apartment I shared with Chris in Chicago; it took us days to figure out what it was.) I steeped the Chinese root in boiling water and gagged it down to no effect. I meditated. Oh, did I meditate. None of it helped.

At my first annual checkup in two years (my health insurance coverage was spotty), I saw a new primary care physician. The waiting room of his office was small and painted a disquieting shade of Easter-egg blue. The plan was never to tell him what I'd been experiencing, about how riding the subway made me feel like someone was drilling into my nervous system or how insomnia had become an abiding part of my life.

He was short and middle-aged and brought to mind the word *clement*. His expression was pleasant, his manner confident, giving the impression that none of his patients stayed sick for long. He had a paternal manner and seemed genuine.

We went through the usual pokes and prods. He listened to my heart and lungs and then asked if I had any health concerns.

It didn't seem worth it to tell him. What would I say? *I feel edgy*? *I'm splintering*?

When the exam ended, he left the room, and I dressed. He knocked and came back in to see if there was anything else I needed.

I told him about the edginess though not the splintering.

This evoked an enthusiastic nod. "Sure," he said, going to his prescription pad. After scribbling on it, he handed me a prescription for a medication I'd never heard of: diazepam.

"What's this?" I asked.

"Valium," he said.

I must have looked worried.

"It's like having a glass of scotch."

With the prescription in my pocket, I stepped out onto Fifty-Sixth Street. It seemed harmless enough to fill it. I'd keep the Valium around, just in case.

———

That night in my apartment, I stood in the kitchen. The translucent orange prescription bottle sat on the counter. On the radio, a reporter talked about the US occupation in Iraq.

Deciding I didn't need to take a pill, I went back to bed. I lay there for hours. The edginess grew into a tormenting, low-level hum in my chest. I breathed in-and-out, in-and-out.

The hum swelled. My mind started on repeat: *I can't take this, I can't take this, I can't take this*. This wasn't like the hypochondria. Hypochondria had staying power. It was a slow preoccupation; this was splintering from the inside out.

I got out of bed and paced. My apartment looked out onto the Brooklyn–Queens Expressway. Cars zoomed by, too fast. The tormenting hum swelled again, breaking, flooding me with mute horror.

Turning on the kitchen light, I filled a glass with water and fumbled with the Valium bottle. Finally negotiating the top off, I tipped the little blue pills into my hand. *A whole or a half? Two?*

Then came the thought, *You're just being dramatic*—a phrase so often thrown at women. I was *being hysterical*. I didn't want to *be hysterical*. After funneling the pills back into the bottle, I twisted the cap closed.

———

I hadn't been told my diagnosis, but I hadn't asked either. He may have assumed I was there for the Valium. The diagnosis was a formality.

Valium was one of the first "wonder drugs."[15] There'd been others—Thorazine for psychosis, lithium for mania, and Elavil and Nardil for suicidal depression—but those were for the "insane." Valium was "mother's little helper," a "happy pill" for housewives.[16] (Miltown was the happy pill of the 1950s and SSRIs for the 1980s and 1990s and 2000s and 2010s and . . .) As a remedy for everyday stress, it changed psychopharmacology. Drug companies didn't need to develop medication for people with severe mental illnesses anymore; they could cater to those who wanted to feel "normal" and "happy" and had the means to pay for it.[17] By the 1970s, it was the most frequently prescribed drug in the United States.[18]

Given the ubiquitous ask-your-doctor and talk-to-your-doctor advertising campaigns, did it really come as a surprise that my doctor might have thought I just wanted a pill? The now seminal ask-your-doctor marketing ploy started in 1976. The manufacturer of the then prescription drug Robitussin, A.H. Robins Company, came up with the idea. A commercial told viewers, "The makers of Robitussin ask you to ask your doctor." They figured out that they didn't need to sell cough syrup; consumers sold it to themselves and their doctors endorsed it.[19] Today, the US is one of only three countries in the world that allows direct-to-consumer advertising for psychotropic medications. By 2016, pharmaceutical companies were spending nearly $6 billion on direct-to-consumer ads encouraging us to self-diagnose and self-medicate.[20]

What did I expect? Like most physicians, he was trained to identify and treat patients as efficiently as possible with the appropriate treatment, which usually meant a prescription medication. I didn't know it then, but I'd soon learn that talking to a doctor about a mental health condition is like going to a lemonade stand and saying you're thirsty; you're going to get lemonade.

On one of my last days at the school, I saw Jackie in the hallway. She waved for me to wait. As we walked, I heard a clicking sound. At first, I thought it was her high heels ticking against the linoleum floor, but it was the Valium in the pillbox in my pocket. I hadn't taken one yet but carried the pills around with me—five, just in case.

She held open the door and said to let her know if I needed anything.

The smell of bleach hit me as I entered the classroom. I said hello to Ms. Madelyn and Sam and Maria and the students. Kemal greeted me with a *you-talkin'-ta-me?* As I put down my bag and pulled out the handouts, the edginess turned to splintering.

I stood at the front of the room. The edginess came first. Then the splintering inside my mind. I didn't feel capable of reading a poem. It seemed impossible. I asked the students to imagine a machine that could produce love: "Would it be pocket-size? Would it be enormous? What would the love it makes look like?"

The room seemed to fall away for a moment. "Draw a picture of the machine," I said.

Shaky, I passed out markers and the handouts I'd brought. They started to draw.

After circling the room, wishing the class would be over, I walked behind Noel. He'd drawn a television set with wings. It was so animated, so alive. He'd written something, too. I leaned in to read it.

He cupped his hand over one ear, the other over his mouth.

I should have stopped, backed away. Not thinking, I asked, "Can I see your paper?" and picked it up without waiting for him to respond.

He gripped his ear more tightly.

I realized what I'd done. "I'm sorry." I put the paper on his desk.

His face reddened.

"Here." I patted the paper. "It's right here."

If I described what Noel did next, it would make him seem "crazy." My rendering of how the other students responded would make it more so. M. Remi Yergeau, an academic and author with autism, and others write that our "typical autism essays" and gimmicky fiction and irresponsible screenplays about autism silence neuro-atypical people with autism who are better able to tell their own stories.[21] My version of events wouldn't give his perspective.

I'll say this much. Mr. Sam approached him. Eventually, he guided Noel out of the room. Eventually, Ms. Madelyn clapped to call the students to attention. Eventually, the students clapped in response.

Ms. Madelyn suggested we wrap up for the day. I collected the students' papers and gathered my things. As I walked out of the room, the pills clicked in the pillbox in my pocket.

———

Later, I sat on a bench in Socrates Sculpture Park on the bank of the East River. It was once a landfill that artists and neighbors had turned into an outdoor art exhibition. All around were sculptures: the head of a yak carved out of stone, an inflatable Buddha floating in the river, Christo-esque drapes of blue fabric suspended above steel poles.

I pulled Noel's drawing from my bag. On his paper, above the TV set with wings, he'd written: *Draw a picture of the machine.* Why had I taken his paper the way I did?

In its rhetorical form, the question mark is about self-inquiry. It's a way to resolve doubt, a way to cross-examine ourselves. A debate with the self. The self questioning the self.

In English, it appears at the end of a sentence. It requests and inquires. It's our most intimate form of punctuation. It's us at our most vulnerable. It's how we ask for help.

When it serves as a comma in a list of questions, it signals persistence: *Are you tired? Hungry? Angry? Sad?* The desire to know.

According to lore, the ancient Egyptians placed the symbol on maps to mark new and unknown locations. Why that particular shape? Why the lengthening curve? The symbol makes sense when you think of the ancient Egyptians' love of cats. (When a beloved cat died, they shaved their eyebrows in honor of it.) A question mark is the shape a cat makes with its tail when it's surprised or curious.

The question mark may have started in Rome, arising out of the Latin word for question, *quaestio. Quaestio* was shortened to *qo*. Someone, somewhere, wrote the *q* over the *o,* the *q* lost its shape, the *o* collapsed into a dot, and the question mark was made:

$$quaestio \rightarrow qo \rightarrow \overset{q}{\underset{\circ}{}} ? ? ?$$

Others believe an eighth-century scholar named Alcuin of York originated it. His *punctus interrogativus* told monks to raise their voices in question at the end of a clause. The shape first appeared in medieval texts as a dot and a tilde, or "lightning strike," that may have evolved into the mark we know today:

$$\cdot \sim \quad \cdot{\scriptstyle\sim} \quad \cdot ? \quad ? ?$$

The question mark creates a relationship. We use it to ask of one another, to get to know each other—or at least try.

A wind swept over the river. The inflatable Buddha undulated on the waves. The doctor's voice sounded in my ears: *It's like having a glass of scotch.*

I pulled out the pillbox and popped it open. The pill felt light between my fingers. Chalky. Just chalk.

It was insubstantial on my tongue. I sipped from my water bottle and swallowed. After too long, the edginess smoothed out. My mind dulled. A not-unpleasant weakness took hold of the lower half of my body. What was the harm in that?

6

Cracked

The knife blade rested on the grapefruit's yellow skin. Paul stood behind me. He'd asked me a question. My hands shook as I guided the knife through the center of the grapefruit's pink flesh until it split open.

"Out of the blue," Paul said, shaking his head in confusion.

I'd asked him to move out of the apartment we'd shared for half a year. Half a year without conflict. Half a year during which he, an actor—who really was an actor, not trying to be one—had raised enough money to make the feature-length film he'd dreamed of, and I'd produced a poetry festival in Lower Manhattan. (Years later, I'd see his character get stabbed on an episode of the hit TV series *The Americans* and feel unreasonably sad.) Nothing romantic had sprouted between us. No rift had occurred.

"I don't understand," he said. "I've met your mother."

She'd come to visit a few times, and I'd performed well. I'd performed well the weekend my father visited, too. Telling them—or anyone—hadn't been an option, not because I thought they wouldn't be supportive but because I'd grown distant from them and myself. And I couldn't say, *Something's wrong, but I don't know what it is. I'm not—*

I traced the knife along each of the grapefruit's segments. Its juice seeped onto my fingers. Even with the Valium, I wasn't sleeping much. I worked three jobs and completed the work due for my MFA program, all while feeling like my mind was in shards and my nerves were being pulled out of my skin.

Paul stood behind me, waiting.

Such an unreasonable urge—to scream. He couldn't have understood that I needed to be alone—not alone in the sense of the only one in the room but alone as in no one and nothing anywhere ever, so I could stop from breaking or go ahead and shatter completely.

"Well, if you're not going to say anything." He went to his room and closed the door behind him.

The loft—my loft—was in an industrial building not zoned for residential use. It seemed—in my jagged, ramped-up state—reasonable to lease a loft illegally and build it out. I paid for it with the money I earned as a writing consultant in the public schools. I was still a writer-in-residence and had started teaching creative writing for a nonaccredited continuing-education program for adults. The consultancy paid more in a month than I made in a year. A recruiter had seen me teach a class of fourth graders (regular education) at a school in Queens, and the company hired me to mentor teachers and give workshops about how I taught writing, which fit the company's model.

Paul was the first roommate-applicant I'd met with. As soon as I met him, my decision to offer him the second room was made. It wasn't just that he was clean-cut and clearly could pay his rent. He was one of those people who wanted to make the world a better place. With sincerity, he spoke of the book he was reading about stopping world hunger or his passion for LGBTQ+ rights.

He was kind and generous. There was no reason for the tension between us—no reason, except that I was cracking.

I put the knife onto the counter. The Valium was in a pillbox in my pocket. The pills didn't rattle, but their silence had become a kind of call. I couldn't take one yet. It wasn't time. I never took them in the morning before teaching.

At the table, I sat. The need to scream started to fade. Shakily, I ate the grapefruit, licking the sweet, bitter juice from my fingers.

The term *nervous breakdown* wouldn't have occurred to me then. That was something out of the 1950s, when businessmen had too many two-martini lunches, and McLean Hospital was where poets like Sylvia Plath and Robert Lowell went to recover from artistic collapses. Use of the term is said to have peaked in the United States around 1940.

The condition that had also been called a *nervous disorder* or *nervous illness* had been around for almost a century. Someone with a nervous disorder didn't exhibit psychosis (hearing voices; talking to people who weren't there; intense paranoia; speaking in "word salad," where phrases and clauses jumble together nonsensically). A nervous disorder was characterized by exhaustion, mild depression, mild anxiety, bodily complaints (chronic pain, insomnia, irritable bowels), and obsessive thinking. It was separate from "insanity" and most often experienced by the worried well.

In 1869, the neurologist George M. Beard referred to nervous exhaustion as *neurasthenia*, which, he believed, only the elite in society suffered from.[1] It was all the rage among elites, artists, and leaders, as if they alone were prone to the stresses of contemporary life and the sweeping technological advances of the age, like the steam engine. Those afflicted included Henry and Alice James, Edith Wharton, Jack London, and Charlotte Perkins Gilman—whose short story "The Yellow Wallpaper" is a harrowing depiction of the "rest cure" that forced women to isolate in bed and do nothing, a treatment that (unsurprisingly) could lead to psychosis.

My nervousness wasn't from stress, and I wasn't exhausted. My experience was closer to the nineteenth-century German understanding of neurasthenia: an illness marked by a complete breakdown of the psyche.

Later that morning, in the South Bronx, I walked from the "6" train, passing bodegas and men on park benches, toward the school where

I was teaching. The men stared at me—out of boredom or interest or both. Each step I took was accompanied not by anxiety but fragility—fragility fueled by the certainty that I was about to crack.

If I could have a Valium—just a nibble. A "nibble" entailed gnawing off chalky bits of one of the blue pills. A nibble "didn't count." I stopped outside the school entrance. In my bag was a bottle of water and in my pocket, the pillbox. It would be easy enough to—

The doors to the school swung open and a man—an administrator—came out. He nodded. I nodded back, business as usual.

In the foyer, I handed the security guard my bag. He gave it a cursory glance and gestured for me to pass through the metal detector. The bell signaling the change of classes rang. Students poured into the hallway. They shouted. No lockers opened and clanged shut. They weren't allowed to have them, something about them supposedly storing drugs.

I passed a bulletin board half-full of quizzes on display to commend students for getting nineties and ninety-fives out of a hundred. The other half had been ripped off and lay on the floor. The clock on the wall was stopped at 8:42.

When I reached the classroom, I peered in the small window in the door. The eight male students were seated at small desks positioned far enough from each other so that no student could land a punch on another without getting up. Technically, they were in the seventh grade, but they read on a fourth-grade level. A few of them, big and bulky with the beginnings of manhood, looked much older than twelve and may have been fourteen or older and had been held back several grades. They barely fit in their desks.

I'd taught students with their diagnosis before: severe emotional disturbance (SED). One veteran teacher I'd worked with, Ms. Jackson, was fierce and brilliant. Her students had been labeled SED. She said that although they didn't behave, they weren't "emotionally disturbed." They were angry. "They're smart as hell and have never been taught to read or write. They've slipped through the system. Wouldn't you be angry?"

Students with SED were challenging. In a different classroom, at another school, during a heated argument over a notebook, a student had yanked another student's hair so hard she pulled her to the floor. Once, a student threw a desk across the room. Twice, I'd been spit at.

Classroom management, in many ways, was out of my control. I was just a visitor. The teacher set the tone.

As I entered, the head teacher, who sat at her desk, looked up and clicked her chin as if checking me in. Then she went back to eating Oreos. The assistant teacher sat on the other side of the room at her desk eating Doritos. If she noticed me, she didn't show it.

Two students in the back row stared out the window. Two in the middle row—leaning toward each other, low and obvious—passed something between them. One in the front row quietly stared down at a book, reading, as if in a different classroom where learning actually took place. Darnell sat slumped in his chair with his arms crossed.

On one of my first days, the teacher had complained to me—loud enough so the students could hear—that they could "barely read a word." I'd found that five of them could read, albeit with difficulty. It had taken seven of my ten classes with them, but those five had eventually allowed me to see what they could do.

Darnell hadn't given me the chance. He never looked me in the eye. Once, when I stood at the front of the room trying to teach, he muttered—loud enough for me to hear—"White bitch." With the other students, he was wry and funny with a charm that bordered on charisma.

As I passed the first row of desks, Darnell slumped lower in his seat, muttering a loose, "Shi-yit."

The teacher called me over. She leaned forward as if to whisper something to me. Then, loud enough for everyone to hear, she said, "Dar-nell has a pro-blem."

Darnell grimaced and looked away.

"We had a visit from a nice man from the zoo. He brought reptiles for the children to learn about." She addressed Darnell. "You want to tell her what you did?"

Darnell clearly didn't. My participation in this public reprimand wasn't going to strengthen our relationship. I went toward the board to start the lesson.

"Dar-nell," the head teacher went on, "grabbed one of the frogs, took it by the mouth, and tried to *rip* it in half." I kept writing on the board. "In *half*," she repeated. "Which is why he'll be leaving us soon for his VIP appointment with the vice principal."

Darnell continued to look away. There was a flush to his cheeks. I couldn't tell if it was embarrassment or anger or both.

There came a knock on the door. A man poked his head in and called Darnell's name. Darnell rolled his eyes and slunk out of his chair. He walked so slowly that the man had already stepped into the hall and the door had closed. I expected Darnell to open and slam the door shut, but he didn't. He just let it close behind him.

I handed out six different translations of Bashō's haiku — *The old pond / A frog jumps in: / Plop*. I told them that each of them would read it in his own way. They were decidedly unimpressed. I'd taught them Shakespeare, Langston Hughes, Etheridge Knight, and Sylvia Plath, and none had moved them to anything beyond groaning participation.

During the mini lesson on imagery and haiku, I entered what I called the teaching zone — snatches of time when I wasn't splintering or I wasn't thinking about Valium. My mind was centered. My body felt strong. Barely managing to keep their attention, I went over how a haiku was three lines and followed the syllabic count of 5–7–5. (Japanese doesn't translate syllabically into English that way, but the syllables make it easier to teach.)

I assigned them to write their own. They twisted in their desks as if being physically tortured. When I reminded them that they only had to write three lines, they perked up. One jibed the student next to him: "You can't even write one line." Soon, they were all ribbing each other until they were competing to show who had written the most lines.

———

The majority of them had been subclassified with oppositional defiant disorder. (At the time, confidentiality either wasn't followed or didn't exist because I shouldn't have known their diagnoses.) ODD first appeared in the DSM-III as oppositional disorder, which said that a child between the ages of three and seventeen who exhibits two—*two*—or more of the following over six months was pathologically antisocial: (1) throws temper tantrums, (2) violates minor rules, (3) argues, (4) displays provocative behavior, or (5) is stubborn. Don't most children—and many adults—throw temper tantrums? What child doesn't violate minor rules? Isn't stubbornness a requirement of anyone under the age of thirty?

The DSM-III-R attempted, in its own feeble way, to limit the number of children diagnosed with ODD by adding the word *often*: often throws temper tantrums, often violates minor rules, etc. But "often" was such a vague measure as to be useless. The DSM-III also added more symptoms, bringing the total to nine, including "often swears" and "deliberately annoys people."[2] It also eliminated the safeguard that the child had to be older than three to be diagnosed (terrible twos, anyone?).[3]

The DSM-IV did little to help.[4] It lowered the number of symptoms to eight, removing swearing but leaving in "argues" and "deliberately annoys people," and reinstated the minimum age of three. Again, it emphasized "clinical significance."[5] As with adults, "clinical significance" doesn't determine if a child's behavior and thinking are extreme enough to be pathologized. It sounds scientific, definite, but in practice means little. Darnell's actions and mental state were "clinically significant" if he demonstrated one—just one—of the following: an inability to learn not explained by other factors; difficulty maintaining relationships; or inappropriate behavior, moodiness, or fears associated with school or personal problems.[6]

The DSM-5 hadn't yet been published, but it wouldn't have helped Darnell escape a diagnosis either. It left the ODD diagnosis basically unchanged and introduced the highly controversial disruptive mood dysregulation disorder, the crossover symptoms of which—irritability and temper tantrums—made it possible to diagnose more children with both disorders.[7]

The ODD diagnosis invites so many sexist and racist assumptions and implicit biases as to border on unethical. ODD primarily stigmatizes children of color. A 2010 study states—openly and in writing—that disruptive behavior disorders like ODD are predictive of "later criminal charges."[8] Couple that stigma with a study that showed that clinicians are more likely to diagnose young people of color with ODD.[9] Add to that the multiple studies that demonstrate how children of color receive stigmatizing diagnoses like ODD whereas white children are given a (relatively) less stigmatizing diagnosis like ADHD. Had Darnell been white, he may not have received a diagnosis at all. In one review, researchers found that the behavior and emotional states of young people of color are pathologized with what are widely considered to be more serious mental illnesses.[10]

Having received a diagnosis like ODD and entering the mental health system, Darnell would likely remain in it, encountering racism well into adulthood.[11] Studies have shown that physicians' implicit biases are major factors in determining a diagnosis.[12] Latinos are three times more likely to be diagnosed with psychotic illnesses than whites are.[13] Blacks are nearly twice as likely as whites to be told they have schizophrenia.[14] Native and Alaskan Native patients have the highest rate of psychiatric diagnosis and are most likely to report mental distress, yet whites receive the most services.[15] This disparity has been found in marginalized communities overall.[16]

(Rates of diagnosis according to race and ethnicity are controversial. Some say people from racial and ethnic minority groups don't have an increased risk for psychiatric disorder but that mental illnesses in marginalized groups are more persistent.[17] The "persistence" of mental illness could be the result of barriers to care and systemic racism: lack of insurance and access to providers, cultural and racial insensitivity, and the unavailability of economic means to pay for care.[18] Most researchers agree disadvantaged racial and ethnic minority groups are less likely to have access to and receive treatment, and others argue it's because blacks, Native peoples, and Latinos tend not to report to mental health care providers due to stigma, religious beliefs, lack of diversity among providers, language barriers, distrust in the health care system, or lack of insurance.[19])

The ODD diagnosis begs many questions: How often are black boys deemed "aggressive"? How much more frequently are black girls perceived as "resentful"? Aren't the rules associated with behaviors like tantrums and emotions like anger and argumentativeness determined by the dominant (white) culture's norms? Who decides if Darnell's stubbornness is clinically significant? A white school counselor or therapist?[20]

Unlike Darnell, I wasn't a child caught in a system loaded against me. I had the privilege to ignore whatever diagnosis the doctor had given me so I could fill my prescription of Valium and take the little blue pills now and again—and again and again.

———

On my way home on the "6" train, I sat in the nearly empty subway car and tried to read Emily Dickinson, whose poetry I loved and didn't understand. Her use of dashes—not the crosses and other calligraphic oddities—drew me in (*I heard a fly buzz—when I died—*). Though critics made much of how she used them—for emphasis, to introduce a list, to interrupt, and as parentheses—no one knows what she meant in every instance. To me, they function as place markers, a way to guide the reader beyond normal punctuation. They also usher the reader through—inviting us to keep reading.

I fingered the pillbox in my pocket. At Eighty-Sixth Street, people piled on. I gave up my seat in case someone needed it more than I did. A white man in a business suit took it. Oblivious to the pregnant woman next to him, he sat and stared down at his magazine.

At Lexington, more people got on, forcing me to the back of the train. A woman pressed against me. The Grand Central stop brought more people. As they squeezed in on me, I tensed as the cracking feeling took hold.

A pill—just one.

I pulled out my pillbox, elbowing the woman behind me as I did. I unzipped my bag and grabbed my water bottle. It was empty. I hadn't filled it before leaving the school. Nimbly, I popped open the pillbox with one hand, raised it to my lips, tongued a pill, and swallowed it dry.

When I got home—soupy from the Valium—Paul was out. On the kitchen counter, he'd left a note saying he wanted to talk. I didn't want to talk; I wanted another Valium.

————

The next afternoon, I went to a professional development meeting for my consultant job. Inside a small auditorium in an elementary school on the Lower East Side, I sat with the other consultants and listened to my Australian supervisor talk about accountability frameworks and a balanced literacy approach. The cracked feeling returned. *You have to get out of here—or take a Valium—just one, a nibble.* If I hadn't had to teach a creative writing class that evening, I would have.

That night, I sat at the head of a circle of desks in a classroom in a West Village elementary school rented out by the continuing-education company I worked for. Around and across from me sat my four students: an MBA grad, a stay-at-home mom, a librarian, and a waitress, all of whom wanted to learn to write fiction. The librarian loved romance novels and hoped to publish one someday. The MBA student read John le Carré and imagined a series of his own. The waitress read and wrote raunchy experimental fiction that made me feel like a puritan. The stay-at-home mom wasn't sure what she wanted to write.

We were studying characterization in a short story by Jhumpa Lahiri. I brought up punctuation—not in the story but in general. I asked if they ever thought about how expressive parenthetical marks could be. "Commas," I said, "are like two speed bumps that barely slow the reader down. Parentheses (almost always) force the reader to step inside. Dashes—always—elide and invite the reader in."

Two of my students seemed to brace themselves. Another looked away. It had been the same in my MFA program. Punctuation and grammar barely got a mention, as if writing had nothing to do with them. Never mind that my fellow MFA students, like these uncomfortable students before me, didn't know how to use commas or dashes or parentheses, let alone any of the more sophisticated punctuation marks like the semi-colon, with any kind of style. Punctuation, supposedly, made students nervous and hampered their creativity. I never understood how aspiring writers could expect to feel at ease and inspired while writing if they didn't know how to punctuate sentences.

At the end of class, my students stood—smiling and talking of the characterization assignment I'd given them. I wished them good night. As I put on my coat, the pills rattled in my pocket. I'd forgotten about them. Maybe I didn't need them, after all.

I practically strode down Sixth Avenue. But by the time I reached Twelfth and Second, the fragile feeling crept in. It was too much: too much noise, too many people, too many cars, too many lights.

At the sound of a car honking behind me, I turned. My neck cracked. I pulled my water bottle from my bag and took two Valium.

———

Later I learned that Valium's risk for addiction is extremely high. The more I took it, the harder it was for my brain to function without it. Valium has a longer half-life than other benzodiazepines like Xanax, Klonopin, and Ativan. The onset of action is rapid, it peaks after an hour, and then lingers for up to two days. Dependence is quick. Withdrawal produces the same symptoms it's prescribed to treat: anxiety, insomnia, panic attacks—and worse—psychosis, seizures, suicide.[21] Valium activates dopamine in the brain, which may help in the short term.[22] It also hijacks the reward system, causing it to malfunction. The need for more increases. Memory and learning are affected.

I could fault my doctor and the pharmaceutical drug industry for putting me at risk, but I couldn't have held those little blue pills in my hand without a diagnostic code. My primary care physician might have written *300.02*, for generalized anxiety disorder, on my chart. Having a diagnostic code made it possible for me to pick up my schedule IV narcotic from the pharmacy and for him to be reimbursed by my insurance company for my visit.

If I'd known he'd labeled me *300.02* and that meant "generalized

anxiety disorder," I might have believed him. My mother always said I
had a "singular way" of worrying about the world. On a routine visit to
the doctor, I supposedly sat on the examination table while we waited
and pointed to the Band-Aids and gauze and sharp instruments on the
counter and asked, "What are they going to do to me that I'm going to
need those?"

Originally, diagnostic codes were supposed to aid in compiling
statistical data and hospital admittances, but their main function has
become helping doctors get paid and patients receive treatment. The
Mental Health Parity and Addiction Equity Act says mental health
benefits should be equal to other medical benefits, but an insurance
company will only cover "medical necessity." That gets tricky when it
comes to DSM diagnoses.[23] Is treatment for what are considered more
minor diagnoses, like anxiety, medically necessary? Psychiatrists, psychologists, and others use "workarounds," labeling patients with false,
more severe diagnoses to make sure that insurance companies will
cover treatment.[24] A doctor who levels a diagnosis may not actually believe the patient even has it. Sometimes, the patient is in on it, agreeing
to accept a more severe diagnosis in return for medical coverage. Even
if the patient doesn't actually believe the diagnosis, it's on the patient's
record and, in a sense, it becomes real.[25]

Even without knowing my diagnosis, my prescription marked me.
If I'd seen a psychiatrist and told him I was taking Valium and it had
helped—which it had in a dark, dislocating, soupy way—that doctor
likely would have seen my prescription as confirmation of a diagnosis. A code like *300.02* was on my medical record. I had a diagnosis,
whether I knew it or not.

———

The following week—my last day at the school—Darnell wasn't in class.
The teacher told me he'd been expelled for the incident with the frog.

"Rightly so," she said, loud enough for the students to hear.

On the board, I wrote a summary of the day's lesson. The students
sat listlessly. Darnell's desk sat empty.

After school, on my way to the train, I thought of how I'd never see the boys in that class again. What would happen to them after having been pathologized as pre-criminal and emotionally disturbed and disruptive at such a young age?

I got home to the loft to find Paul's stuff gone—all of it. He'd moved out that day. Gone was most of the furniture, which had been his. Without a couch or a coffee table or even a light, the loft was dark and bare. Rain collected in a puddle on the floor. Either he or I had left the window open. Most likely—definitely—it had been me.

———

No one knows the true origins of the dash. Some credit the twelfth-century Italian scholar Boncompagno da Signa, who developed his own system of marking punctuation in a text. He used a vertical slash (/) to signal a pause and a horizontal one to indicate a full stop (—). By the eighteenth century, novelists like Samuel Richardson and Laurence Sterne were using it to isolate phrases of unnecessary information or parenthetical asides. (*The pills were there—weren't they always?—and they'd become necessary.*) In the nineteenth century, Charlotte Brontë used them to indicate interrupted speech. She and other authors also used it in aposiopesis, where a sentence is broken off and left unfinished. (*I said the pills were—*)

The em dash—so named because it's about the length of an *m*—primarily connects or interrupts phrases and clauses. An en dash—which is about the length of the *n*—is for numbers, dates, and time: *2000–2007.* The short hyphen connects words and prefixes: *anti-anxiety medication.*

Too often, the em dash can be a way to cut off. To end.

It can also elide. In the US mental health system, people of color are disregarded. Drug research focuses on white men; in some trials, whites make up as much as 90 percent of subjects. The 1993 National Institutes of Health Revitalization Act required drug companies to include people of color, but a 2014 study found that fewer than 2 percent of more than ten thousand cancer clinical trials focused on a racial or ethnic minority.[26] People of color—and children of color like Darnell—exist between dashes.

———

After Paul moved out, the loft felt damp, as if the rain I'd sopped up had stayed. Maybe it was the soupiness of the Valium. The loft felt empty, too, probably because it was. When I spoke on the phone with my mother or my father, which was rare because I'd isolated myself from them and everyone else, my voice echoed in the unfurnished emptiness of Paul's absence. I'd closed the door to his vacant room, but it hadn't helped.

The night I decided to stop taking Valium I was in the bath. The water was warm; the apartment air, very cold. I lifted my hand from the water. Steam rose off it. As the water dripped, I realized that maybe it wasn't normal to keep the thermostat off even though it was freezing. My soupy mind had been saying not to bother.

I stopped taking the little blue pills—just like that. No doctor supervision, which I later learned was dangerous and could have led to seizures or worse. No Narcotics Anonymous.

Insomnia tormented me. Intense stomach cramps sometimes made me double over. My migraines were blinding.

The cracking feeling intensified. I walked the streets to try to lessen it. When it was too cold or rainy, I paced my loft in the near-dark. Out my window, I could make out the Williamsburg Bridge and Lower Manhattan. From Ground Zero, two spotlights beamed into the night sky in memory of those who died on 9/11. In the building next door, a television set flickered blue, faded, and flickered blue again.

One night, I walked the Manhattan streets until after midnight. Down one block and the next. I let the stoplights tell me which way to go. At a walk sign, I'd cross; don't walk meant turn the corner.

I repeated the few lines of a Dickinson poem I could still recall:

I cannot live with You—
It would be Life—

And Life is over there—
Behind the Shelf—

I reached Astor Place, where a man and woman were spinning the Cube. I turned around and headed back uptown, through Union Square to the New York Public Library.

The lions on either side of the library glowed in the spotlights. The scene made me think of old New York and *The Great Gatsby* and Fitzgerald's essay "The Crack-Up." In "The Crack-Up," he talks about breaking down and becoming little more than "a cracked plate." His situation was nothing like mine—and I felt nothing like a plate—but the cracking was the same. The essay had one of my favorite lines in it, which I never got quite right: ". . . the test of a first-rate intelligence is the ability to hold two opposed ideas in the mind at the same time, and still retain the ability to function."

I stared at the lions' stone faces. To me, it seemed unlikely that Darnell had intended to kill the frog. It also didn't seem plausible that he tried to rip it in half "to get attention," as the teacher had said. It had to be more complicated than that. Maybe a storm of anger had come over him and the frog was part of that storm. Maybe he hadn't considered that what he was doing might inflict pain. Maybe he wanted—

I had no idea what Darnell wanted. As a white, privileged woman with Valium in her pocket, I didn't pretend I could.

———

A notice arrived from my landlord. The building had been sold. Because it wasn't zoned for residential, I was technically a squatter who happened to have spent thousands building out her loft. They gave me a month to move out.

I started to cry—then sob. In the kitchen, I took the pillbox from where I'd stashed it in the cupboards behind the herbal tea. Three little blue pills left.

I fumbled to get the pillbox open. Then I put it on the counter and called my mother. All I could muster were scattered words. "I—I—"

My mother said, "Try to calm down."

"I just—"

"Take a breath," she said.

"I—"

"Take a breath."

I kept stuttering—my words broken off by dashes.

Weeks later, she came to New York to help me pack. It was clear—even to me—that living in the city wasn't working anymore. When I opened my apartment door to greet her, she didn't say anything. I must have looked as shattered as I felt. She tried to cover her reaction with a hug.

We sat on the floor wrapping dishes in newspaper and talked about what would happen next. I didn't tell her about the Valium. I said I just wanted to take a break from New York, put my belongings in storage, stay with her in Chicago for a while, and then come back.

She wrapped a knife in newspaper and nodded, unconvincingly.

"I mean, I have to come back. I need to—"

"We'll see how it goes," she said.

7

Doctor's Orders

At my mother's, I did the dishes and vacuumed and dusted and cooked to try to make up for worrying her. She said she was happy to have me there. It seemed hard to believe.

We didn't call it a nervous breakdown. Or depression. We didn't call it anything. My father, stepmother, sister, and brother-in-law weren't aware of what was happening. My niece and nephew were too young to wonder why Aunt Sarah lived with Nana while other adults had their own houses and families.

I didn't tell my mother how much pain I was in. In what had once been her study and was now a makeshift room for me, I cried—quietly, so she wouldn't hear. It was as if leaving New York had flipped a switch on my tear ducts.

To try to crawl out of the spiral I'd fallen into, I walked the same route day after day. I did a thousand downward dogs. I taught creative writing online, which, except for my mother, was the extent of my social life. That year and a half is a series of snapshots: me at the desk in "my" room, writing articles and essays about literature; thick, insomniac nights staring out the window at the lights in the apartment building across the street; me deplaning in Madrid to interview the novelist Javier Marías for *The Paris Review* and then in Tokyo to interview Nobel laureate Kenzaburō Ōe; my byline in the *New York Times* and

then *The Atlantic*; applications to graduate school; my acceptance letter to the doctoral program in English literary studies at the University
of Iowa.

The need to leave my mother's came on fast. Part of me must have
thought that if I stayed with my mother too long, it would mean I had,
officially, cracked. Surely, six years in a PhD program would pull me
out of it.

Iowa City seemed perfect. Named the UNESCO City of Literature, it was the bastion of reading and writing I'd thought I'd find in Seattle. It was also a cheap place to live, which made it seem like buying a
house was a good idea. I cashed in my IRA and all my savings and took
the money my mother and father and stepmother generously gave me
to buy it. It turned out that my meager teaching assistantship barely
covered my mortgage payments and living expenses.

But being in the program was like being on an idyllic, inconsequen-
tial planet made of books. It made me feel removed and sheltered. My
department spoke a different language: dialectical materialism, the
Lacanian Symbolic, *langue* and *parole*, double consciousness, Foucaul-
dian semiotics, heteroglossia. I was exempt from "real life" and spent
my time happily alone researching in the stacks (in a real library with
actual books) or reading in a café or writing papers at home. Occasionally, I attended a reading or a department party, which made my social
life seem vibrant.

It was a life of the mind. I was quiet and calm. The edginess—the
splintering, the cracking—was gone. I was solid, whole. Feet on the
ground. No longer in a spiral. At least that's how it seemed.

———

One afternoon, at the end of my fourth semester in the program, the
students in my Interpretation of Literature course sat in their desk
chairs arranged in a semicircle facing the board. The course was a
general-education requirement few would have opted to take. We'd
finished *Wuthering Heights* and they'd submitted their final essays, so I
did a creative assignment with them.

I wrote on the board: *Free write about uncertainty.* They weren't creative writers—most were business majors or premed—and looked at me as if to say, *Really?* I smiled. They humored me. They always humored me, mainly because I'd promised the course wouldn't be a waste of their time and had made good on it. They wanted practical skills. I respected that. Almost all of them—at least the ones who'd done the assignments—said they were leaving my class more confident in their writing, which, I told them, would make their lives exponentially easier.

They pulled out their spiral notebooks and pens or opened their laptops.

"Ten minutes," I said, looking at the clock. "Go."

After class, I went to my office and sat at my desk to grade their final essays. My rubric tested them on one punctuation mark only: the comma. I'd learned that six of the ten most frequent writing errors people made involved commas. If I taught the students to use commas correctly, they'd be *that person* in their workplace: the "good" writer. I gave presentations on comma rules, quizzed them, went over the rules again, quizzed them again. Some were curious from the beginning. They'd never been taught grammar or punctuation. Some wanted to keep it that way.

I pulled out the stack of final essays. The first was written by one of the few students who hadn't paid attention, barely came to class, and had failed all the quizzes. I scanned it: commas like he was decorating a Christmas tree. I thought of Mr. Baker and my tenth-grade term paper. With my blue pen (most students had been scarred by years of red ink telling them how wrong they were), I circled the first error.

When I finished grading, I went home and slumped my bag, heavy with the latest stack of library books, onto the coffee table. I made myself dinner and sat at my dining room table. The food on my plate was monochromatic: orange. Different shades but still orange: carrots, sweet potatoes, butternut squash. One color—that was the rule.

Many rules had come and gone. I'd eliminated and reincluded foods—ordering and reordering what could be eaten and what must be avoided. Each change seemed vital. Meat was off-limits, no matter how grass-fed; then it wasn't. Fish was permitted but only farm-raised;

then only wild-caught. My nightshade intolerance was confirmed; then it was questionable.

Then I lit on color. Only green foods. Then only yellow. Then only purple and blue. Then only red and white.

The thoughts were intense, particularly if I'd eaten the wrong color: beets and purple cabbage instead of kale and zucchini. My mind looped again. *Purple. No, green. Orange. Green. Definitely green.*

—————

Distress. Disorder. Dysfunction. Disability.

Distress is the result of external or internal pressure (e.g., a tornado, worry). It's a kind of torture. The distressed person feels both constrained and compelled to act. My eating habits were odd but not distressing.

The primary definition of disorder is confusion. One could have argued my food choices were odd. Eating by color—the ROY-G-BIV diet—wasn't yet a thing but within the decade would appear in *Food & Wine* and on the Food Network. But I wasn't confused.

Psychiatry has never been able to define what makes thoughts, emotions, and behaviors dysfunctional. The DSM doesn't offer the equivalent of, for instance, systolic blood pressure numbers to determine if you have stage 1 hypertension or are in a hypertensive crisis. I may have deviated from the norm but I was functioning well enough. I ate. I taught. I did my coursework and passed my exams. I'd traveled to San Francisco to interview the poet Kay Ryan for *The Paris Review* and later interviewed the Pulitzer Prize–winning novelist Marilynne Robinson.

Clearly, I didn't have a disability—or did I? Were my movements, senses, or activities limited by how I was thinking? In comparison to whom? At what point does a person say, *I'm distressed, disordered, dysfunctional, disabled*? How do we judge if the person is right?

—————

My therapist Anne had a deep voice and chin-length hair and always wore jeans. In her office, she sat facing me on one couch; I sat on the other. My grad-student health insurance was good to the point of in-dulgence and almost everyone in my program saw a therapist, so I did, too.

Anne's curtness appealed to me. During most of our sessions, I complained about my "problems"—the pressure I felt about my up-coming exam, difficulties choosing my dissertation committee, uncer-tainties over a grading decision with a student. To most of what I said, she basically told me to get over it. Usually, she was right.

She knew about the anorexia and my drinking and New York and living with my mother but not the suicidal images and thoughts. She never asked about diagnoses or medications. I'd never told her about my monochromatic eating.

That day, for some reason, I did. She asked me how I was doing. Offhandedly, I mentioned my one-color-only diet.

She asked how much time I spent worrying about it.

I asked if that included the hours spent at the co-op shopping for food (I knew almost all the employees by name) and writing up meal plans and cooking said meal plans and checking and rechecking.

She said yes.

I told her.

She said, "You might have OCD."

———

In obsessive-compulsive disorder, the obsession is invasive and relent-less. It's uncontrollable and guilt provoking. The obsessive thoughts are often of doing harmful or repugnant acts. Commonly, they stem from a need for order, symmetry, reassurance, or purity. The obsession is resisted, which is where the compulsion comes in. We often associate OCD with someone who washes her hands. The obsessive thought of contamination arrives and the compulsive action of handwashing alle-viates her distress. When the thoughts return, the compulsion has to be enacted again and again, even though the skin on her hands is splitting open and may be infected from the incessant handwashing.

OCD, in its current form, first appeared in the DSM-III and has changed little. It was categorized under "anxiety disorders" until the DSM-5, when it was filed under "obsessive-compulsive and related disorders." To be diagnosed, I only needed to display an obsession or a compulsion that caused "marked" distress, interfered with my normal routine, or took up more than an hour a day. The research disagrees that the two are mutually exclusive; half of all OCD cases given by primary care physicians are misdiagnoses.[1]

OCD is stigmatizing and disabling. Sufferers aren't laughed with; they're laughed at. (*Oh, that's just my OCD acting up.*) The disorder interrupts their lives, straining relationships and sometimes—though rarely—leading to suicide.

In DSM terms, it was possible I had it: recurrent or persistent ideas, thoughts, images, or feelings (check); the compulsion to act on them (check); psychic discomfort and extreme doubt, which might look like a nervous person (check). I'd already had a classic OCD subtype: body dysmorphic disorder.

I took a *do-I-have-OCD?* quiz online. Did I excessively count and arrange? (Anne seemed to think so.) Examine my body for signs of illness? (Check.) Unnecessarily reread or rewrite? (It was my job.) Avoid colors associated with unpleasant things? (Absolutely.) After just twenty questions, I scored a fifteen: *OCD is likely.*

I called the specialist Anne recommended to make an appointment. The soonest was two months away. I took it.

———

Summer came. I didn't have to teach and was expected to work on my dissertation. As if on cue, distraction set in. I was in the tiny attic of my house at my desk, files open to the notes I was supposed to be taking on the history of phrenology.

The idea of finally writing a profile about Shuvender Sem took hold. It seemed better than trying to write my dissertation. I'd known about Sem for a couple of years. He'd come up in a random Google search I'd done while still living with my mother. The headline in *The Guardian* had read: "Trouble in Transcendental Paradise as Murder Rocks the

Maharishi University."[2] Inset was a mugshot of Sem: hair disheveled, gaze remote, eyes sneering at the camera, upper lip curled as though caught on a hook. During a psychotic episode, he'd killed another student. He'd later been found not guilty by reason of insanity (NGRI). I'd bookmarked the article, thinking someday I might write about him and Transcendental Meditation (TM) and the Maharishi, who'd since passed away and whose devotees had once included the Beatles.

I googled Shuvender Sem again. He was confined to a psychiatric facility two hours from where I lived. He'd grown up in a small town in Pennsylvania? How many Sems could there be? I called information. It took a minute, maybe less, for the operator to locate his family and give me the number. His father answered. When I introduced myself as a journalist (though I'd only written book reviews for the *New York Times*, arts and culture pieces for *The Atlantic*, and done interviews for *The Paris Review*), Mr. Sem sounded impatient. He asked no questions, just for my phone number. I gave it to him. He said he'd get back to me and hung up.

Ten minutes later, my phone rang. A recorded voice told me I had a call from the Independence Mental Health Institute (IMHI) in Independence, Iowa. Sem came on the line. He introduced himself as Shubi.

"You're a journalist?" he asked.

I said I was interested in interviewing and writing an article about him.

Without prompting, he told me about himself—how he'd grown up in Pennsylvania and had his first psychotic episode at seventeen or eighteen. He and his father hadn't always gotten along. And then: "You ever read Thomas Friedman? The columnist?"

I said I had. I was about to ask what he liked about Friedman when he said, "I gotta go. My card's running out." The call ended.

———

References to schizophrenia date back to ancient Egypt and India. Kraepelin referred to it as *dementia praecox* (no real relation to the dementia we know today) but by the end of his career doubted the validity of his diagnosis, writing that schizophrenia might "not represent the expression of particular pathological processes, but rather indicate the areas of our personality in which these processes unfold."[3] In 1911, Eugen Bleuler (who also lent us the term *autism*) reframed it, calling it *schizophrenia* to describe the patient's "split mind"—split from reality, not among personalities or between parts of the self. (There has been ongoing debate if Bleuler actually thought a patient was split from reality or split between parts of the self, using *schizophrenia* as a synonym for dissociation; most, however, agree that it does not refer to "split personalities."[4]) Both Kraepelin and Bleuler characterized schizophrenia by psychosis: hallucinations (seeing things that aren't there) and delusions (believing things that aren't real). During the early twentieth century, neo-Freudians blamed it on a patient's overcontrolling "schizophrenogenic mother."[5] Other psychotherapists blamed it on the family.

Throughout the DSM's editions, definitions and categorizations of schizophrenia changed.[6] The DSM-I called it *schizophrenic reaction* and included seven subtypes: simple, chronic, catatonic (in a stupor), paranoid, schizoaffective (which seemed to overlap with mood disorders), childhood, and (the condemning) residual (when a person no longer has an acute "schizophrenic reaction" but shows what they called *residual disturbance*). The DSM-II removed *reaction*, calling it *schizophrenia*. Though the DSM-III acknowledged that nongenetic factors would be as important as genetic ones, it conceived of the disorder as something that labeled a patient for life.[7] In its attempts to order and sort and reclassify, the DSM-III renamed it *schizophrenic disorder* only to change it back to *schizophrenia* in the DSM-III-R. The DSM-IV tightened the diagnosis by stating that a patient needed to display acute psychotic symptoms for at least a month, up from the DSM-III's one week. (Both editions specified a patient needed to show signs of the illness for at least six months but disagreed on the amount of time that "active-phase symptoms" must be present.) The DSM-5 invented a "schizophrenia spectrum," the rate of misdiagnosis and overdiagnosis of which has caused serious concern.[8]

Shubi had killed a fellow student while in a psychotic state. Hallucinating and paranoid, he chose Levi Butler. They'd met only one or two times and had casual conversations, but Shubi had believed he was the head of a conspiracy against him.

————

For weeks, while waiting for Shubi to call again, I researched the murder. Shubi had already been diagnosed with schizophrenia. According to the lawsuit filed by the estate of Levi Butler against Maharishi University of Management and Shubi's own account, Shubi had been paranoid since the day he arrived on campus, believing the CIA had him under surveillance and that a microchip in his brain told him what to do.[9] It's possible that the way he practiced TM exacerbated his symptoms, which meditation can do to someone with a fragile mind, particularly with a history of having been diagnosed with schizophrenia.[10] The result was psychosis and the fatal stabbing of Levi Butler, a veritable stranger to Shubi. (In that same lawsuit, the estate of Levi Butler asserted that the university had "negligently failed to properly screen Sem before allowing Sem to attend MUM and receive TM instruction . . . because MUM employs a two-step admission process, it could be inferred that MUM recognizes that not all students are suited for MUM's TM curriculum.")[11]

Shubi was found NGRI for first-degree murder.[12] The ruling meant that at the time of the murder he'd been insane—a legal term, not a medical one—and couldn't "appreciate" that what he'd done was wrong. He was committed to IMHI for an indefinite period.

I didn't get many calls, so when my Nokia cell phone finally rang, I ran to the kitchen and answered. The recorded voice said it was from IMHI. Shubi came on the line. He had a lot to say, he said.

I grabbed a notebook and pen and sat at the dining room table.

He asked if I knew about everything.

"Not everything," I said. There was a long pause. "Are you still there?"

"You know Melpomene?" he asked.

"Um, a bit."

"The muse of tragedy."

"Okay," I said.

"Tragedy," he said. "I mean, when I talk to you, aren't you like, 'Shit, this is such a sad story'? Sorry about the language. Isn't it? Your readers will think so, too. They're bound to. I mean, I'm sane now, you know? I make my own decisions. And I'm taking classes."

"That's great." I pressed the tip of my pen to the paper.

But he didn't talk about the murder; he told me about a puppy his parents had bought him and how he'd been living at home because college hadn't worked out and he'd been arrested and hospitalized and homeless in Philadelphia—where he'd learned which shelters were safe and which food pantries had the shortest lines and what time each served which meal—and then was hospitalized again and put on crazy drugs that made his head feel like "it was going to explode" and how he'd searched the internet and found MUM's website and interpreted it as a promise that TM would make him better and would disconnect the microchip in his brain, so he visited the campus and then went there, but he kept getting worse and the black cat started following him.

I waited.

"Yeah, well, I gotta go. My card's running out."

And he was gone.

———

Midsummer, after we'd had similar calls, I asked if I could visit him in person. He hedged for a while—not calling—but finally agreed. After filling out the forms and getting permission from his psychiatrist, Dr. Z, I drove to Independence.

IMHI was more elaborate than I'd imagined. Pine trees and box elders bracketed the grounds, secreting the building from the main road. When the building came into view, it was straight out of *Jane Eyre*: domes, corner towers, barred attic windows. It had been built in the nineteenth century as part of the "Kirkbride plan," created by the Quaker physician and mental-health advocate Thomas Story Kirkbride.

Kirkbride designed structures to improve the inhumane conditions in insane asylums across the country. At the time, serious mental illnesses basically fell into two categories: *insanity* and *idiocy*, though the terms were often used interchangeably. Kirkbride insisted people with mental illnesses could be cured but needed fresh air, beauty, privacy, and comfort. The center structures of his buildings proudly faced out and the wings let in fresh air and natural light. They housed museums, libraries, and workshops. Patients had their own rooms, which had twelve-foot ceilings. They sometimes tended the lush grounds themselves. Mental hospitals, Kirkbride said, should impress the patients and inspire faith in the psychiatric profession.

IMHI was one of only a few Kirkbride buildings that hadn't been torn down or abandoned. During the 1960s and 1970s, following John F. Kennedy's push to close all psychiatric facilities and replace them with community centers, many were demolished or abandoned. Kennedy meant well, but deinstitutionalization failed miserably. It was supposed to be the answer to the inhumane treatment in psychiatric facilities, where patients had once been chained to walls, left unclothed and sitting in feces, subjected to ice baths and, later, lobotomies, forced sterilizations, straitjackets, and overmedication. The idea was that community centers and prescription drugs would be enough to care for people with severe mental illnesses. Under Kennedy and Lyndon Johnson and Jimmy Carter and all the presidents in between, the number of Americans receiving treatment in mental hospitals dropped by 70 percent.[13] Patients were sent "home" though few had one. Those in need of long-term care were forced out with nowhere to get help. Most of the promised community centers never opened and mental health funding was slashed until people with mental illnesses were living on the street or in jails, receiving inadequate or no treatment. Chicago's Cook County Jail became one of the three largest mental health facilities in the country, along with Los Angeles County Jail and Rikers Island.[14]

Inside, IMHI wasn't quite as grand. Paint peeled off the walls. The tile floors were scuffed. The reception area was chilly, almost cold. The only sound was the buzz of fluorescent lights and the bluster of the air-conditioning system. That and the *tick, tick-tick-tick* of the receptionist's keyboard. She had me fill out more forms and told me that my point of contact—Dr. Z—would be with me soon.

When Dr. Z entered the reception area, he quickly extended his hand and introduced himself. He had a determined mouth and soft eyes. His blazer was threadbare along the lapel. After we shook hands, he spun on his heel and walked out.

I followed him through a series of wide corridors. He slowed and said that, originally, he hadn't wanted Shubi at IMHI. "We don't have violent offenders here."

Most people with mental illnesses aren't violent. Studies show that statistically they are no more likely to be violent than anyone else.[15] According to the US government, only 3 to 5 percent of violent acts are carried out by them, and they're ten times more likely to be victims of violence than people without mental illnesses.[16] The tendency toward violence has a much higher correlation with a history of substance abuse and domestic violence.

Dr. Z led me up a stairwell. A cage blocked the shaft, ostensibly to prevent patients from falling or attempting suicide.

We reached a door marked *Residents' Lounge*. He held it for me. The room was crowded with men mostly—young and old—seated on couches or sitting at tables. It smelled of urine and bleach. Only a trace of Kirkbride remained: through the arched windows came an almost honeyed light.

On one couch sat a boy wearing a bike helmet. Arm's length from him was one of IMHI's aides, a robust man wearing a white uniform. Each time the aide tried to take the boy's hand, the boy coiled away from him.

At the sight of us, the boy perked up and came toward us. His bike helmet tilted to one side of his head, making him appear disheveled and a little stylish. Drool dangled from his chin. When he was near, I realized that he wasn't a boy but a man. He asked me if I wanted a blowjob. I said, "No, thank you." At this, he seemed satisfied and headed back toward the couch.

A chubby patient wearing a T-shirt that read *My other car is a*

Rolls-Royce meandered around the room, cradling a juice box in his hands. Through the tiny straw, he took slow sips.

Dr. Z showed me to a table and told me to wait. I slung my bag over the back of the chair and sat. The residents' lounge was nothing like the one portrayed in *One Flew Over the Cuckoo's Nest*—certainly not the theatrical movie version with Jack Nicholson wide-eyed and wild and the patients on the ward each a stereotype of mental illness (the novel, written from Chief Bromden's point of view, is quieter and has more depth)—but it was chaotic. Many would have said disorderly, definitely abnormal.

After he'd gone, I pulled out my notes to review. During this time, thoughts burst through (*orange, purple, green*), but I was so focused on Shubi that "my OCD" (I'd already started to believe I had it and that it was part of me) seemed to have gone away. Was it possible for OCD to just disappear? What about schizophrenia?

———

The anti-psychiatry movement of the 1960s and '70s questioned (1) if mental illness was real and (2) if psychiatrists had the expertise to tell us it was.[17] Many factors triggered the "movement" (it wasn't a single organized group): forced treatment, involuntary commitment, the extreme effects of drugs like Thorazine, the biases and prejudices of DSM diagnoses (e.g., homosexuality), and the dehumanizing treatment in mental hospitals and asylums. It was made up mostly of academics and theorists, not practicing physicians: Michel Foucault, Gilles Deleuze, Felix Guattari, Erving Goffman, Thomas Scheff. They critiqued psychiatry from perspectives analyzing patients' rights and state power. Some in the movement saw diagnoses like schizophrenia as methods of social control, a way to criminalize those considered different or deviant.[18] To those in the anti-psychiatry movement, the "mentally ill" were an oppressed group and psychiatry the oppressor. R. D. Laing, a psychiatrist who studied psychosis and has been associated with the anti-psychiatry movement, said they were exceptional beings; others said prophets.[19]

Though some set out to enact reform, others wanted fame and to shame psychiatry. David L. Rosenhan's "Thud experiment" caused the biggest stir. In the early 1970s, he and seven volunteers supposedly went into psychiatric institutions and pretended to hear the words *thud*, *hollow*, or *empty* to be admitted. In his report "On Being Sane in Insane Places," which was published in 1973 in the prestigious journal *Science*, he declared psychiatry "cannot distinguish insanity from sanity."[20] Rosenhan's study had none of the investigative flair of Nellie Bly's exposé of the asylum on Blackwell's Island in the 1880s or the integrity of Erving Goffman's book on St. Elizabeths Hospital in the 1960s, both of which set out to show the conditions of mental hospitals. Rosenhan's study was more of a trick. (Ironically, though most fail to point this out, it proved reliability among the clinicians: all but one of the "pseudo-patients" were diagnosed with schizophrenia based on the same symptoms.) Ultimately, all he did was show that even if a patient lies convincingly about having psychiatric symptoms and says he needs help, an admitting physician in a psychiatric hospital will probably believe the patient and try to help him. The study was later alleged to be deeply flawed. According to an extensive book by Susannah Cahalan, Rosenhan falsified data and blatantly lied.[21]

Like all DSM diagnoses, schizophrenia has no known biological marker. It can't be tested the way cancer or Parkinson's can. Said to be chronic and with a dismal prognosis,[22] it's often seen as the most disease-like of all mental illnesses. Psychiatrists and researchers insist that genes and environmental factors play a role.[23] But so far, no one has been able to prove what it is or isn't.[24]

In *The Myth of Mental Illness* (1961), psychiatrist Thomas Szasz (who insisted he wasn't part of the anti-psychiatry movement though he's almost always associated with it) argued there was no such thing as mental illness. In a stab aimed at biological psychiatry, he wrote that mental illnesses weren't diseases because diseases existed in the body and mental illness was found in thoughts and behaviors. Mental illnesses weren't even illnesses because illnesses exist only in terms of how a condition deviates from the norm and no "norm" has ever been established in psychiatry the way it has in other branches of medicine, where strep throat—a bacterial infection—is evidenced by inflamed (abnormal) tonsils. "Normal" in psychiatry is laden with moral and prejudicial judgments about how people *should* think and act; instead, Szasz argued that mental illnesses often came from "problems in living."[25]

Szasz went so far as to say that people "play" mentally ill. Szasz, of course, was a theorist, not a researcher, and cites no studies. (He spends an entire chapter on "metalanguages" and philosophies of signs and signifiers and symbols that would have made the linguist Saussure proud.) His own practice was brought under suspicion when, in 1992, Szasz was sued by the widow of a patient who killed himself after Szasz was said to have convinced him to go off his medication.[26] Unlike others critiquing psychiatry, his arguments focused less on psychiatrists as oppressors and patients as the oppressed; psychiatry simply wasn't a legitimate medical field.

Szasz would have opposed Shubi's NGRI sentence. To him, criminal behavior was never the result of mental illness. Had he learned the details of the murder, Szasz might not have been so quick to judge. Or if he'd been in IMHI's residents' lounge with me. If Szasz had been there and insisted that the young men around us were faking or weren't ill, I would have said he was crazy.

———

Dr. Z returned with Shubi in tow. Shubi seemed to drift. He was fleshy though not fat. He wore a well-ironed button-down striped shirt tucked into a pair of creased baggy jeans. His cheeks bulged, and the shocking bald spot on the crown of his head made him appear much older than in his twenties. The dark circles under his eyes spoke of a life spent primarily indoors.

When he stood at the table across from me, I extended my hand. "It's great to meet you."

He gazed past me out the window. "Long drive?"

"A bit," I said.

He lowered himself onto the chair across from me. When we were both seated, Dr. Z settled at the table, giving us space without affording us any actual privacy. I pulled out my MP3 player and pressed *record*.

I said something about how the profile was going to be great and thanked him for meeting with me and asked what he wanted from it.

"For people, especially the Indian community, to understand that I'm not just some schizo and a murderer."

A group of patients entered the lounge. A young man, his face dominated by a pair of puffy lips, noticed Shubi and called to him. Shubi waved and continued talking.

I let Shubi wander from topic to topic. He described at length the day he filled in the drainage holes on his family's property with dirt, causing the toilets and sinks to back up, because one of the voices in his head told him to.

He told me about the time he spent in the county jail before being tried. "I was on suicide watch. That's how bad off I was right after. They wouldn't let me have anything but a blue blanket. It can't be folded. Or tied. No sheets. Just a blue blanket."

"That must have been hard," I said.

"Do you get along with your father?" he asked.

I thought of how little I spoke to my family. My father had visited me in Iowa the previous year. We'd spent the day planting the flowers that now bloomed in my yard. I'd brought out a portable stereo and as we dug in the dirt together, we listened to a recording of Hemingway's "Hills Like White Elephants." Then I made him a dinner—this was pre-color—of sautéed white fish and steamed broccoli. He'd eaten the broccoli and asked, "How does this taste so good?" I told him I'd made it with love.

Shubi shared a long, disjointed story about his father's army service in the Sino-Indian War. I glanced at Dr. Z, who looked bored, like he'd heard it all before.

The man in the bike helmet weaved toward us again. When he reached the table, Shubi said hello. Then the man wandered off and curved back around in the direction of the couch and the aide.

"That's Jerry," Shubi said. "My roommate. He and I—we live together. I sort of take care of him."

I asked how he learned TM.

He glanced at Dr. Z.

Dr. Z stood up. "Why don't we walk outside."

The rest of my visit was spent meandering the grounds, listening to Shubi tell stories but nothing about the murder.

Dr. Z briskly showed me out. I drove back to Iowa City, alongside trucks barreling down Interstate 380, past cornfields and abandoned farms and vacant silos, over Paha ridges—those Grant Wood, *American Gothic* hills—hoping Shubi would call and I could still get his story.

———

Weeks later—the night before I was to see the OCD specialist—my phone rang.

Shubi said hello. "Some days, I end up curled in a ball on the floor. That's how bad I feel about what happened." Long pause. "Someday, I'll be out of here, and I'll have a girlfriend." Another long pause. "That's why I can't let this thing mess me up."

"What thing?" I asked.

"This thing with you," he said.

"The article?"

He said his lawyers had told him not to talk about the murder.

"I understand," I said, wondering if he'd ever intended to tell me.

"I gotta go. My card's running out."

He ended the call.

In the attic, I filed the reams of court documents and put away my notes. A few times, I thought I heard the phone ring. It was his story to tell.

I went outside onto my porch. Morning glories hung from the trellis. The stillness was palpable. The chirping crickets could barely be heard.

One thought came and then another. *Green. Orange. Green. Definitely green.*

The morning glories' blue petals were cupped closed. They seemed mute, but they'd open again in the morning.

———

The apostrophe is the one punctuation mark that indicates possession — what we own, what's ours. *Sarah's OCD*. *Shubi's schizophrenia*.

It's not a popular punctuation mark. People typically list several reasons to abolish it: (1) it's confusing, (2) it's unnecessary, (3) James Joyce didn't use it in *Finnegans* (no apostrophe) *Wake*, and George Bernard Shaw called them "uncouth bacilli." (Shaw didn't actually have anything against apostrophes. He was a savvy businessman, who wanted to make money by selling the print versions of his plays and believed that his unique page design — typeface, margins, paper, binding, and, yes, quirky punctuation — would help him sell books. Apostrophes were only "uncouth bacilli" when they didn't fit with his aesthetic design and eccentric printing requirements.)

The apostrophe was meant to help us clarify, but its rules aren't always logical. Some scholars suggest it came into being during the transition from Old to Middle to Modern English: *the kingses madness* became *the kings his madness* became *the king's madness*. Unfortunately, it's not as simple as just adding an apostrophe and an *s*. With singular words that don't end in *s*, few stumble — *Shubi's crime* (the crime belongs to Shubi) — less so if the word ends in *s*. Generally, words that end in *s* — singular and plural — get only an apostrophe: *the girls' disorders* and *the species' diseases*. Exceptions involve names (biblical and otherwise), sibilance, letters, and acronyms. And then there's the pronoun issue: *it's* versus *its*, the contraction of *it is* as opposed to something that belongs to *it*. *Theirs*, *hers*, *yours*, and *ours* also get no apostrophe.

Although we think of the apostrophe primarily in terms of ownership, the word comes from the Greek for "to turn away" — maybe because taking possession of one thing means letting go of another.

———

The next afternoon, on my way to the OCD specialist, I walked through town, passing students in Iowa Hawkeye T-shirts. The sky clouded over, then turned an ominous green. Iowa had profound rainstorms. A sky that green usually signaled a tornado.

Dr. W wore tortoiseshell glasses and was mostly bald. His mustache was bushy and hung over his lips. I'd looked him up on the internet. His research was on compulsive gambling and obsessive behaviors present in personality disorders.

We sat. He asked me questions. I answered. As I did, he often brushed his mustache with his index finger, a distracting gesture that seemed a bit compulsive.

He asked if anyone in my family had OCD. I said no. He asked if I was on any medications. I said no.

"Not that you would be—if you had OCD," he said. "People with OCD tend not to be open to taking pills." He paused, brushed his mustache. "For fear of being poisoned."

I sat up straighter. "Does medication work?"

Another pause. Another brush of his mustache. "About 60 percent of the time. Though if you ask me, that's a generous estimate. Most patients' symptoms are relieved by cognitive behavioral therapy."

"Is that what you recommend?"

He raised his eyebrows. "For you?"

"Yes."

"You don't have OCD."

We'd only been talking for ten minutes.

"Look," he said. "Sometimes, the diagnosis—or lack thereof—is clear." He brushed his mustache and said my concerns about food were limiting and "not ideal" but not debilitating.

"What do I have?"

He shrugged. "I can refer you to a colleague."

I left his office and walked across the bridge. The sky had grown darker. It seemed to me that his offer to refer me to a colleague meant I had *something*; I just had to find out what it was.

As soon as I was home, rain started to tap against the roof. Tiny taps. In the kitchen, from the fridge, I pulled out broccoli, a bunch of curly kale, and zucchini and placed them, in all their green, on the counter. I laid the cutting board beside them.

The wind picked up outside, whacking open the neighbor's fence. As I started to chop garlic, the outdoor tornado alarm sounded. I put down the knife. In the basement, I crouched beside the stairs, turned on my emergency radio, and waited to be told when it was safe to return.

8

Treatment/Options

What came next is hazy: me at the table on my back porch next to the hydrangea bush my father planted; an empty wineglass in front of me; other half- and quarter-full wineglasses on the table; a plate of half-eaten crackers and cheese reminiscent of a cocktail party; two men stepping through my back door into my house, one calling over his shoulder for me to hurry or I'd be late for the reading.

I must have followed the two men—poets I'd become sort-of friends with—into my house and out the front door. I remember the three of us walking down the sidewalk in the early-autumn night air. It's possible I tripped over a crack in the sidewalk because my palm was scraped when we reached Dey House and entered the reading room. The author at the podium—whoever it was—didn't hold my attention. I sat in my chair with all the other mostly want-to-be writers in the room and thought of how drunk I was and how great it was that no one could tell.

It had been that way for weeks: glasses and glasses of wine meant to stun my thoughts into submission. They moved so fast I could barely keep up with them. (Racing thoughts, by definition, *race*, meaning they move at a rate faster than can be expressed in speech. They zip through, barely touching our consciousness, communicating to us without us knowing.) Unrelenting, they left me full of enough worry and regret and anxiety to start drinking again.

But alcohol only made my racing thoughts harder to track and more unreasonable. It also lessened my inhibitions. I started wandering the streets at night, like I had in New York. I had sex with a visiting professor an hour after meeting him. I made promises to myself not to drink. Then I'd sit at my dining room table to prep for teaching, get up for "just one glass," and wake up in a near-face-plant on a book.

Only my hangovers brought relief. I didn't care about the nausea and dry heaving and headaches. A hangover could slow my thoughts or shut them out, at least temporarily.

The one time I taught a class hungover I stood at the front of the room staring into the faces of the students in my Interpretation of Literature class. For fifteen minutes I lectured on the second chapter of Robert Louis Stevenson's *The Strange Case of Dr. Jekyll and Mr. Hyde*. The point was to set up how Stevenson's use of multiple points of view prevents us from understanding Dr. Jekyll, the novel's protagonist. As I spoke, I forgot a minor character's name. Twice, my stomach turned and I thought I might throw up. When I finished, a student raised her hand and reminded me that (as the syllabus I'd written myself stated) they hadn't started the book yet.

I went into my office and cried, less because I'd made a fool of myself than because my hangover was wearing off and my thoughts were again becoming belligerent, urgent, unrelenting.

Weeks later, I had my annual checkup with a new primary care physician. I sat, hungover, on the examination table. The familiar white paper crumpled under my thighs. My thoughts raced, occasionally colliding with my hangover, leaving me soggily on edge.

Dr. B was tall—almost looming—and thin. His ears were remarkably long. His scraggly beard and thick-rimmed black glasses made him seem a little scatterbrained but devoted.

After the exam, he pushed up the sleeves of his white coat. Did I have any concerns?

I mentioned not sleeping well. "And my thoughts are all over the place. I can't concentrate."

Without a pause, he nodded. "ADHD." His tone wasn't authoritative, just matter-of-fact. Under the cool fluorescent lights, he said I needed a stimulant: Ritalin. We'd titrate up to determine the right dose.

I left the hospital and walked across the bridge with the Ritalin prescription folded in my pocket. After I filled it and returned home, I went to the kitchen and put the pill bottle on the counter. Maybe I did have ADHD.

In a way, it made sense. Of course. What I'd thought was OCD (hypervigilance, obsessive thoughts, social isolation) was ADHD (hyperactivity, overfocus, social isolation). ADHD seemed harmless, almost normal. In a college town like Iowa City, it was hard to meet someone who didn't have ADHD.

I filled a glass with water. The white pill was tiny between my fingers. I put it on my tongue. Almost tasteless, it was easy to swallow.

———

It's hard to explain exactly what a thought is. The definition is circular. A *thought* is "something that a person thinks." Other definitions approximate it: "a mental formation, effort, or activity." Its synonyms are equally abstract: *idea, consideration, notion*. Current scientific thinking suggests that a thought is a chemical reaction in our brains—a millisecond signal from one nerve cell to another via a synapse.

Most agree that a thought is fleeting. The number of thoughts we have per day is debated. The "fact" that we have sixty or seventy thousand thoughts per day is vastly overstated. Most recent studies approximate six thousand. Few thoughts have the staying power to become a belief—a truth we live by.

———

A year or so later, the prescription bottle of Ritalin sat on my kitchen counter. By then Ritalin was an integral part of my life. My day was dictated by my morning dose, afternoon dose, and evening dose (if needed, which it always was).

I popped open the lid, thumbed a pill, and took it with water. The drug seemed to take a split second to work. In reality, thirty minutes had to pass before the methylphenidate seeped through my stomach lining, into my bloodstream, and found its way to my brain, where it raised my dopamine levels[1]—releasing feelings of pleasure—and harmonized my neurons.[2]

Soon, I felt attentive—distraction-proof. I went to my office in the attic and pulled the yellowish three-ring binder off the bookshelf. Flipping past pages of handwritten notes and charts and journal entries and timetables and daily schedules highlighted in yellow and pink and green, I reached that day's entry. On top was my "prefrontal checklist" and "thought-capture brainstorm" of what needed to be done that day. My color-coded planner broke down larger tasks into smaller ones. In the margin, I'd jotted "popcorn thoughts" that had come up while I was trying to work. I kept a food journal. (I'd quit drinking the day I started the Ritalin. It seemed obvious: If I was sick enough to take a psychiatric medication, I was too sick to drink alcohol, a depressant, or take recreational drugs, which I didn't anyway.) Dr. B said my diagnosis was chronic; I'd have ADHD for the rest of my life and had to manage it. So I managed it.

There were moments when I doubted the diagnosis. The classic symptoms of hyperactivity and inattention didn't really apply to me (*high energy* and *intense* were more accurate). But ADHD was different in adults: the criteria hadn't been created for them and so were often applied more loosely.[3] In the adult-ADHD classic *Fast Minds: How to Thrive If You Have ADHD (or Think You Might)*, I found evidence for almost every symptom the authors listed: forgetful (sure), achieving below potential (of course—I hadn't gone to an Ivy League college and isn't that the measure?), stuck in a rut (I'd been drinking), time challenged (who has a great relationship with time?), motivationally challenged (no, but I could let that one go), impulsive (yes, sometimes, when the impulse took me), novelty seeking (I wasn't drawn to find out what that meant), distractible (not at all, but the authors and the internet said this symptom could be replaced with hyperfocusing, which seems different, but I let the contradiction stand), and scattered (not really, but sure). Plus, when I told my mom, she said she could see it; I'd always been hyperactive as a child.

As I worked at my desk, a warm vibration started at the top of my skull. My mind seemed to narrow. I grabbed a yellow highlighter and marked where I'd gone off schedule that day: the thirteen minutes I'd gotten sidetracked while doing laundry, the sixty-eight minutes I spent walking instead of grading my students' essays. My heartbeat quickened. Then it started to pound. Sweat pooled under my arms. Soon, the familiar high-pitched whir inside me began.

Ritalin made me extremely efficient. All the clichés applied: *laser-focused*, *on it*, *dialed-in*. It offered me a tunnel where the more extraneous of my six thousand racing thoughts couldn't enter.

The years of resisting medication were over. No *maybe/maybe not*. No taking a day off as Dr. B suggested and no concern that I might become dependent on Ritalin or that it was making me worse. The tiny white pills had been prescribed for *my* mental illness, *my* diagnosis, *my* ADHD.

After writing my dissertation for three hours with barely a break to use the bathroom and make a cup of coffee (caffeine gave the last of my short-acting Ritalin a bump), I went downstairs and stared out my living room window. An early-summer evening light cloaked the street. My head started to pound. When the short-acting Ritalin stopped, "Ritalin rebound" hit hard: headache, nausea, heavy sadness.[4] I accepted it as part of my diagnosis.

––––––

One of the most dismaying aspects of DSM diagnoses is the way psychiatric medications are used to convince patients that they do indeed have a mental disorder. The medication-as-proof-of-diagnosis theorem is the diagnostic equivalent of *if the shoe fits, wear it*. Because DSM diagnoses can't be proven, medication is said to confirm that the patient does, in fact, have the diagnosis. The effectiveness of the Ritalin supposedly meant I had ADHD.[5] Of course, Ritalin has the same effects on someone with the diagnosis as someone without it.

The flaws in this are twofold. One, taking a medication doesn't mean you have the illness it's said to treat. By this logic, I should also have had narcolepsy, which Ritalin is prescribed for as well. Two, psychiatric medications can create positive, or at least desired, effects in someone without a mental illness. A person without ADHD or any other diagnosis can take an amphetamine like Ritalin and experience an increase in energy and focus.

I'd also fallen prey to the better-than-the-other-medications fallacy: A medication seems effective when the other medications tried are intolerable.[6] Finding the right medication and the right dosage had taken months. We'd tried short-acting and long-acting versions of Ritalin and other pills like Adderall, which made my throat feel like it was closing, and Concerta, which made my muscles stiff to the point that I could barely sit up in bed. Even if the Ritalin rebound was brutal, the side effects of the Adderall and Concerta had been so awful I believed it was perfect. The troubleshooting (*either/or*, never *if*) proved Ritalin was the right medication, which proved it was working, which proved I had ADHD.

Another disturbing aspect of DSM diagnoses is that primary care physicians (PCPs) aren't adequately trained to diagnose psychiatric conditions. A 2000 survey found that PCPs received a median of thirty-two hours of psychosocial training over the course of their residencies.[7] That's the equivalent, in terms of time, of bingeing on a few seasons of the medical TV drama *Grey's Anatomy*. In 2011, a survey reported that some medical students receive less: eight weeks of interview training the first year and eight weeks of inpatient units the third year.[8] The third-year training is often with the most severe cases requiring hospitalization, not those of us who might mention symptoms that sound like depression or anxiety during a routine office visit.[9] Program directors of medical schools around the country admit to this. From 2001 to 2002, a majority stated that their mental health training was "minimal" or "suboptimal."[10] (Since then, many have called for improvements to the curricula but no widespread changes have taken effect.)[11] I'd accepted my primary care physician's diagnosis without knowing any of this, not once thinking he didn't have the expertise to diagnose me with ADHD or prescribe me Ritalin.

Dr. B had likely filtered me through the lens of his experience, that of a primary care physician in a college town. He prescribed me Ritalin based on the symptoms I described (*My thoughts are all over the place*) and the very, very little he knew about me (PhD candidate finishing her dissertation) and plucked ADHD from the many diagnoses the DSM offers. How many of his patients were students complaining of the same symptoms, all being given a diagnosis of ADHD?

––––––

Six months later, the foundation of my house literally collapsed. In one of Iowa's torrential rainstorms, my street flooded. I went down to my basement to prepare for the inevitable water that would pool onto the floor. (When I bought the house, I was told that every basement in Iowa gets water.) I turned on the dehumidifier.

I was on my way toward the stairs when part of the brick wall chipped off. Then a spray of water—like a Roman fountain—burst through. I ran upstairs, grabbed my laptop (priorities), and slipped into my rain boots.

As I stepped onto the porch, there came a crack and then a rumbling sound. I jumped the four front stairs. Wading into the street, I didn't want to turn around to see what the crack and rumbling sounds had been.

The length of the foundation had collapsed, taking with it most of my gravel driveway. The house itself didn't crumble, just tilted as if about to topple. I thought only of my medication. (*My medication.*) I'd left it on the kitchen counter. A guy, a student, probably, came down the sidewalk.

"Please," I said, "I need your help."

I somehow convinced him to walk along my buckled driveway, through the backyard, in through the kitchen window (I'd locked the back door and hadn't brought my keys), across the flooring of my foundationless house, which could have toppled at any moment, and rescue my Ritalin as if it were some sort of helpless cat.

The loss of my house sent me over a new yet familiar edge. My homeowner's insurance covered none of the damage. My father and stepmother paid to fix the foundation, but I was so rattled, so unwell that I ended up shutting them out and seemed horribly ungrateful for their help, for which I was extremely grateful. My mother and sister tried to counsel me, but I was in a shell.

My boss at the Iowa Young Writers' Studio, where I taught creative writing that summer, arranged for me to stay in the university dorms. I sold my house for less than it was worth, just so I didn't have to sleep there again. My furniture, too. My mind wasn't right. I walked the streets of town in a rattled daze.

———

ADHD's history in the DSM is one of loosening and broadening.[12] It first appeared in the DSM-II as *hyperkinetic reaction of childhood* and was characterized by hyperactivity and distractibility. The DSM-III renamed it attention deficit disorder, which could come with or without hyperactivity as a subtype. What was once "hyperkinetic reaction of childhood" need not include hyperactivity. Subsequent editions of the DSM created attention deficit/hyperactivity disorder—with a slash.

As punctuation marks go, the slash seems unimportant, appearing most often in web addresses. It doesn't boast an illustrious history. Also known as a virgule, a solidus, or a stroke, it came to us via Italian rhetorician/scholar Boncompagno da Signa in the twelfth century.[13] Originally, it indicated a pause but by the twentieth century, it was shorthand for *or*, signaling a choice: *yes/no*.

With the slash, the ADHD diagnosis became AD/HD: attention deficit disorder (ADD) or attention deficit hyperactivity disorder (ADHD). The inclusion of the slash created two subtypes: combined, predominantly inattentive (ADD) or predominantly hyperactive-impulsive (ADHD). Subtypes can be used to avoid overdiagnosis, but the inclusion of ADD and ADHD in the DSM-IV made it easier to diagnose, especially in girls who didn't demonstrate hyperactivity, a key symptom in ADHD. As the number of diagnoses increased, principals, parents, and teachers with no training in psychiatry or psychology started to diagnose children, demonstrating how user-friendly the diagnosis was.[14] Drug companies got in on it, too, marketing Adderall and Concerta and other stimulants to children. The result was a false ADHD epidemic, during which, as one study showed, the DSM-IV criteria increased prevalence rates by 64 percent.[15]

The DSM-5 broadened the diagnosis further. It said patients must show symptoms in two settings (home and school/work and home) but required fewer symptoms in teenagers and determined that the age of onset in children only had to be before age twelve, not before age seven.[16] It's unclear how some could call the DSM-5's failure to correct the missteps taken in the DSM-IV a sign that the criteria "withstood the test of time," but some did.[17]

Not that the DSM was solely responsible for my—or anyone else's—ADHD diagnosis; others helped. Pharmaceutical companies enjoyed the most influence but policy makers, politicians, researchers, academics, psychiatrists, nonprofit organizations, celebrities, and the internet had a hand in it, too. Policy makers allowed direct-to-consumer advertising of ADHD drugs on TV, in women's magazines, and on the internet.[18] Politicians looked on when the FDA warned[19] that drug companies were making unsubstantiated claims for those drugs.[20] Academic psychiatrists at universities like Harvard took under-the-table research funding while conducting studies that "proved" the efficacy of ADHD medications.[21] Pharma funded internet campaigns to propogate the erroneous idea that ADHD was a biological disorder.[22] The nonprofit Children and Adults with ADHD (CHADD)—which offers events, webinars, strategies, and resources about the use of medications—was reported to have received nearly a quarter of its funding from pharmaceutical companies.[23] Celebrities like radio host Glenn Beck proselytized the benefits of his ADHD medication on the air. Some of the self-diagnosis quizzes and checklists online were sponsored by drug companies.[24] The media reported and rereported and reported again on the "ADHD epidemic" that never was.[25]

Still, the "epidemic" wouldn't have been possible without the DSM-IV. Although task-force-leader Allen Frances argued that the true culprits for the spate of ADHD diagnoses were drug companies, he also publicly apologized for having expanded the diagnosis: "Our goal was to prevent diagnostic inflation from growing and our conceit was to think we had succeeded in holding the line. We were wrong. It turns out that the impact of the diagnostic system is not in the words as written, it's in the way words come to be used."[26]

Words and (he forgot to mention) punctuation.

––––––

That fall, I was chosen to be the caretaker of an enormous house. The university was starting the Grant Wood Art Colony and while waiting for codes and permits and contracts to be finalized, it needed someone to reside at the home. It was a historical landmark. The artist Grant Wood had lived there in the 1930s and 1940s. One of the professors in my department was on the committee for the art colony. She'd heard about my house and asked if I'd be interested. I said yes and moved into a nearly vacant, five-thousand-square-foot house.

The vaulted ceilings, heated bathroom floor, and majestic claw-foot tub should have been enough. There was also a bed and a desk and an armchair in the master bedroom. The kitchen had a table where I could eat. But the house echoed as I walked. It was so eerie, so unreal that, oddly, it became easier and easier to spend all my time there, alone in only a few rooms, the rest of the house empty and dark.

The racing thoughts were back, even with the Ritalin: *running, food, colors*. Every afternoon at exactly 3 p.m. or 4 p.m., the sodden pit in my stomach returned. And the cracking I'd felt in New York. All of it at once.

I tried every natural treatment I could find: valerian root tea, GABA supplements, tryptophan, lavender oil, a vegan diet, yoga. And meditation—more meditation: Zen, Tibetan, Vipassana. I walked in circles "feeling every step" with Thich Nhat Hanh, searched for my "inner body" with the spiritual teacher (and multimillionaire) Eckhart Tolle, questioned my thoughts with Byron Katie, and mindfully did the dishes as the American mindfulness proselytizer Jon Kabat-Zinn instructed.

Meditation didn't agree with me. Some of the practices produced mild anxiety; others a harrowing, claustrophobic panic. Negative, even severe reactions to meditation aren't uncommon, just not reported in the media. A 1992 study of long-term meditators found that 63 percent experienced at least one adverse effect after meditation retreats.[27] In 2015, a study showed that some subjects experienced negative side effects ranging from anger and anxiety to a psychotic breakdown.[28] A 2017 study documented that 25 percent of people who meditated experienced unwanted effects, including panic attacks and depression.[29] It also reported that many studies on mindfulness-based interventions didn't measure adverse effects and only looked at the benefits of meditation.

One afternoon, I went for a run. Melting snow rushed down the gutter. Puddles formed between chunks of ice. I breathed the cold air in through my nose, into my lungs, and out my mouth in a fog. The sodden pit in my stomach grew heavier, my thoughts more vicious. Dodging the puddles, I ran faster, not caring as I lost my footing on the snow. Once home and inside, I started to sob. The sound seemed so foreign, so strange, it might not have been coming from me.

———

At my annual checkup, I sat in a chair beside the familiar examination table. I was clothed. Dr. B sat beside me typing into the computer.

When he asked if I had any concerns, I told him about the encompassing darkness, the crying spells and bleakness, the harrowing hopelessness, the sodden pit in my stomach, though not quite in those terms.

As he typed, he told me I had OCD.

"OCD?" I thought of Dr. W touching his mustache.

He nodded.

"And ADHD?"

He nodded. "Attention deficit disorder/OCD features with some depressive anxious elements."

I didn't mention Dr. W. He seemed unimportant. Dr. B was my primary care physician.

Dr. B prescribed me an antidepressant. "It will be like wearing glasses," he said. To illustrate, he removed his glasses—which had square black frames and startlingly thick lenses. He faced me. His eyes looked fuzzy. "Nearsighted. I can't see far away." He put back on his glasses, adjusting them so they rested peacefully on the bridge of his nose. That was how it would be for me to take an antidepressant (SSRI). Like wearing glasses. A simple adjustment.

As I stood in line at the prescription counter at CVS, it occurred to me—for a moment—that he could be wrong. Simple, except my adjustment wouldn't be external. I wouldn't be able to remove the pill and its effects at will. My adjustment would be internal, neurological—how permanent I didn't yet know.

But Dr. B was a real doctor. I'd received the diagnosis in a university hospital, not someone's office on Eighty-Fourth Street. And he'd been right about the ADHD. *Attention deficit disorder/OCD features with some depressive anxious elements.*

At home with my new prescription, I stood at the kitchen counter. The SSRI rested in my palm. It was oblong, orange. It smelled astringent, caustic. I placed it on my tongue, where it rested, bitter. I sipped from a glass of water and swallowed it.

Relief—or was it calm?—washed over me.

––––––

If I could go back, I'd ask what the slash meant: *attention deficit disorder/OCD features with some depressive anxious elements.* Either/or? ADHD or OCD? What exactly were depressive anxious elements? Were they optional too?

Dr. B hadn't given me an anxiety test or a depression questionnaire—not that either would have made my diagnosis any more reliable or valid. The most common anxiety test—the GAD-7—and two popular depression questionnaires—the Hamilton Rating Scale for Depression (HAM-D) and the Patient Health Questionnaire (PHQ-9)—don't provide certainty of a DSM diagnosis.

The HAM-D, for instance, doesn't equate to a major depressive disorder diagnosis in the DSM-IV. It wasn't meant to; it's used to prove the efficacy of antidepressants. It asks seventeen questions, but the clinician asks and scores them, determining the severity of each symptom for the patient. I would have done well: depressed mood (check), suicidal thoughts (no), insomnia (100 percent), feelings of guilt (so much—my father, my stepmother, the house), anxiety (I'd like to meet someone on Ritalin who doesn't experience palpitations, stomachaches, sweating, headaches, and have to pee a lot), stomach complaints (sodden pit), difficulty working (no, thanks to the Ritalin), slowness of thought and speech (not even close), agitation (absolutely), hypochondria *(it had returned)*, and "insight" (the recognition that the patient is depressed). The HAM-D is said to have an internal reliability rate of somewhere between 46 and 97 percent, but that comes from studies that only test people already diagnosed with a mental health problem, and clinicians complain that its scoring is "unclear."[30]

As for the PHQ-9, it's steeped in conflicts of interest. Engineered in the 1990s by a group of psychiatrists at Columbia University, the funding came from Pfizer, often referred to as "pharma giant Pfizer," maker of the antidepressant Zoloft. Even the most not-depressed person will register as depressed on it. The nine leading questions give the person few options. The Kafkaesque questionnaire evaluates a patient on a scale: minimal depression, mild depression, moderate depression, moderately severe depression, or severe depression. There is no *not depressed*. The murky gray of *minimal depression* is the best one can hope for. That diagnosis comes with a prescription: "The score suggests the patient may not require treatment." Grammatically, the use of the modal *may* could be a verb tense choice (*might* being past tense, *may* being present tense), but its effect is one of likelihood. There's no implication that the patient *doesn't* need treatment or *might* not need treatment; the patient *may* not need treatment, meaning the patient probably does.

———

It was an unlikely time to fall in love. I must have thought I was well enough to be in a relationship. Ray's dating profile had few pictures of himself, though enough to see that he was attractive; the rest were image after image of his paintings. They were so clearly done by some-one with a singular mind and way of seeing the world. His occupation line didn't read *artist*, but *Finish Carpenter and Construction Superintendent*. He lived in Chicago. A long-distance relationship might work. I was tired of Iowa City and my family was in Chicago and I wanted to see them, so why not visit and meet him?

On our first date, we went for a walk and stopped for tea to get warm. On our second and third dates, I visited his studio and saw his paintings in person. The canvases, thick with paint, were even more vibrant hanging on the walls in front of me. A month later, I met his daughter, Mikka, who was ten and lived with her mother most of the time.

Later, I told Ray about my diagnoses, presenting them as facts. He didn't know a lot about any of the three and didn't care. He loved me. No *maybe/maybe not*.

On weekends, I'd take the Megabus from Iowa and stay with him. Often, in the morning—I'm not sure how I never noticed it before—he couldn't get out of bed. Working construction was so brutal that his joints locked up after he'd been resting. Soon, I'd learn about his chronic back pain, particularly on the days he jackhammered from six in the morning until two or three in the afternoon or worked all night remodeling expensive restaurants.

People love to say there's no such thing as normal, but there is. Although the particulars may differ, normal has a structure. However ethereal, it has a shape. It's solid, consistent, whole. One night while Mikka was staying with us, we went to the neighborhood Mexican restaurant. Ray and Mikka loved each other intensely and battled with the same intensity. Mikka was a tween with reddish hair that curled around her sweetly freckled cheeks. During dinner, she asked Ray if she could finally get a cell phone. Her friends all had them. "Not a chance," Ray said. Pleading ensued. Ray sipped his margarita. "No." Mikka frowned and looked away. Sitting at the table with them, with other families around us, our waiter asking if we'd like anything else and Mikka saying, "Flan," and Ray saying she'd already had enough candy that day, I felt that structure, that solidity, and wanted it to stay.

———

I wasn't with Ray and Mikka the first time the world around me didn't seem real. I was walking down the street in town. Two college-age women passed. They looked at me strangely. I realized my mouth was open and I'd been staring. They didn't seem real. Neither did the bricks I stepped on or the library I passed.

Later that night, at home, I stood before the bathroom mirror washing my face. The stripes on my turtleneck started to blend. I could see through it and my torso. I was disappearing.

By my next appointment with Dr. B, I was certain I was losing my mind. He wrapped the blood-pressure cuff around my upper arm. As he pumped the gauge and it closed around my bicep, my arm felt numb. The room — and he — seemed far away.

"Derealization," he said when I told him.

"And like I don't have a body," I said.

"Depersonalization," he said.

I asked if it was normal.

"It can be," he said, "for someone with your diagnoses."

———

I try to imagine the Swiss philosopher and professor Henri-Frédéric Amiel on July 8, 1880, the year before his death, seated on the stiff-backed chair at his desk. The white in his long goatee doesn't age him. Or it's the plumpness of his cheeks that makes him look so young. But he's aging. It shows in what he writes, his wistful, late-life reflections and inability to remember: "I am *depersonalized*, detached, cut adrift."[31] It's not madness, he says, because madness is the point at which recovering balance is no longer possible and the capacity for self-judgment and self-control have gone. For Amiel, to be depersonalized was a philosophical state, a moment of contemplation.

As a psychological term, *depersonalization*, coined at the end of the nineteenth century, isn't just philosophical *self-strangeness*; it's madness — a pathological state of extreme detachment. One observes oneself from the outside with none of the enlightenment Buddhists with similar awareness claim. Identity and personality dissolve, leaving the person in darkness.

Its counterpart is derealization. The world feels unreal. Time distorts. People and objects drift. Life appears to be simulated.

Hadn't I experienced depersonalization and derealization before? Wasn't that the scrim between me and my classmates on that eighth-grade field trip, the sense of falling away as a migraine came on, the disinterestedness while envisioning my suicide in the bathtub in Chicago, the abandonment present while leaving the hospital after Cappy died, the dark dislocation of living in the Grant Wood House?

———

Diagnoses, plural. If I could go back, I'd tell my thirty-nine-year-old self to slow down. *Consider, for a moment, if you can trust that you have multiple mental illnesses.* I'd tell her that the comorbidity rate in psychiatric diagnoses is extremely high and continues to increase with each edition of the DSM, which could imply that the shifting symptom lists and additions of new diagnoses make people easier to diagnose.[32] My thirty-nine-year-old self might have argued that comorbidity occurs in physical illnesses and is increasing, too. Yes, I'd say, but those illnesses are illnesses; those diseases are actual diseases. They're valid.

Technically, I had one "comorbid" disorder: ADHD and OCD. Only ADHD and OCD were accompanied by codes (314.01, 300.3). My "depressive anxious elements" were a bonus.

Comorbidity—having two or three or four diagnoses—isn't rare. In 2005, a study found that nearly half the subjects had been diagnosed with more than one mental illness.[33] Another study analyzed the frequency of comorbid diagnoses and found that it was "the rule, not the exception."[34] It's not entirely clear if the high rate of comorbidity is the result of inflated diagnoses or a causal relationship among disorders (e.g., anxiety causes depression or vice versa)[35] but given that DSM diagnoses can't be proven, it's not possible to say that one causes another. The move toward multiple diagnoses started with the DSM-III with its abundance of disorders and overlapping symptom lists—a kind of net psychiatry cast to make sure no one slipped through it without a diagnosis.[36]

In some ways, my comorbidity made sense. ADHD and OCD share similar symptoms. So do ADHD and anxiety. And OCD and anxiety. And anxiety and depression. Depression and ADHD are *associated* in that there's much speculation that one causes the other (depression makes you distractible and ADHD is depressing).[37] Once a patient is in the maze of *and* (ADHD and OCD and depression and anxiety) instead of *or* (ADHD/OCD/depression/anxiety), it's hard to get out. The *either/or* factor doesn't come into it.

———

At a water park, on what the brochure referred to as a "monster waterslide," the flimsy, yellow raft beneath me bobbed in the water. Ray and Mikka and Mikka's friend were waiting for me at the bottom. Ray had arranged this trip for us to spend time together.

Lying on my back on the raft, I waited my turn. The boy in front of me in line, his eyes bright with excitement, held on to the side of the slide. I did, too. When it was his turn, he launched his raft forward and disappeared down the slide.

I'd avoided participating in the water park's activities for most of the weekend. I had to work. While Ray and Mikka and Mikka's friend sloshed down waterslides and lolled in the lazy river, I stayed in the hotel room and wrote a book review due to the *New York Times*. It would have been fine if I'd spent the whole time writing, but I also found myself pacing the parking lot for seemingly no reason. Something wasn't right. I was edgy, unable to sit still.

That morning, I'd told them I'd go with them. I wanted to be normal. Stable. Someone with structure.

Which is how I ended up on a flimsy, yellow raft with the girl behind me—bobbing on her own yellow raft—telling me it was my turn. The balding man behind her scowled at me with a *hurry up* nod of his chin. No way back. No options. I let go and drifted toward the slide's mouth.

9

Becoming Bipolar

Ray and I sat at the kitchen table. It was a Saturday morning. We each had a cup of coffee. The French press was between us. Looking bright and happy, like someone bursting with news, he asked what kind of ring I'd want if he were to ask me to marry him.

We'd moved in together, albeit long distance. Technically, I still lived in Iowa. During the week, I taught, staying at the campus hotel, which gave faculty a discount and was cheaper than renting an apartment. On weekends, I paid twenty-five dollars roundtrip to ride the Megabus four hours to Chicago. Ray would be waiting in his gray pickup truck at Union Station when my bus arrived. He'd have on the baseball hat he wore so often I sometimes forgot what color his hair was. (It was blond. He was balding.) As I climbed in, he'd look at me sidelong as if I was the sexiest woman he'd ever met. "Well, hello," he'd say.

I didn't know what kind of ring I'd want; I didn't wear jewelry and hadn't thought about marriage since Chris. Although I'd been socially conditioned in a country where marriage was still very much the norm, I was solitary but well-liked and hadn't kept up with friends and had attended maybe two weddings in my adult life. *Never a bridesmaid, never have to be a bride.*

Children either. Them, I'd sworn off at thirteen when I declared as much to my mother. If I was created only to bear children, as some insisted, that didn't mean I had to do it. Many, many women had assured me I'd change my mind. I hadn't.

But the idea of marrying Ray seemed like a good one. I loved him. I loved Mikka. Being in a stepparent role came surprisingly easily. Basically, I stayed out of it, no matter what *it* was. I deferred to Ray and Mikka's mother. And I understood that although Mikka and I were friends in a stepparentish way, she sometimes wished I didn't exist so she could have her dad to herself.

Marriage was normal. Stable. A structure. If I were married, it would mean I was solid, grounded, not someone who felt herself cracking again.

I had my diagnoses. I had my medications. Never mind that I had to hold myself together all weekend only to sob on the bus back to Iowa. I'd be fine. Everything would be fine.

———

Christmas night at his—our—apartment, we sat on the bed and exchanged presents. A small fake tree stood on the dresser. In the glow of the string of lights, he thanked me for the workout pants and shirts I'd gotten him. He'd never once exercised but had, of late, spoken of it interestedly, like it was an exotic food—live cobra heart or century eggs—he might someday like to try.

After a comedic pause that implied there wasn't a gift for me, he went to the other room. My uneasiness had nothing to do with him. The splintering was accompanied by other symptoms—as I'd started to call them: the cracking feeling, the sense that I was going to break down; the sodden pit, which somehow had taken on the same hue as the murky pit from my teenage years, compounding it. I took my pills. I kept my charts and a calendar and a journal. I did what someone with a comorbid diagnosis with features and elements was supposed to do. It wasn't working.

He came back into the room holding what looked like (and was) a gift-wrapped mop. My stomach didn't sink. My shoulders relaxed. I laughed, genuinely, and pretended to be surprised after I pulled off the wrapping.

"A mop," I said.

From his pocket, he pulled out a Tiffany box. His chronic pain didn't allow him to get down on one knee. He opened the box to show me the ring and asked me to marry him.

It was one of those teasing marriage proposals that winks to the phoniness of the wedding industry and plays with the ridiculousness of what had become a commercialized ritual at best. But there were many reasons to say yes: his fortitude and humor, his talent, how devoted he was to Mikka, and the chance to be Mikka's stepmother.

Solid. Grounded. Not cracking. Yes.

———

We were at Target buying something for the apartment when the shift occurred. Or maybe it had already occurred and the breaking down and cracking had reached a crisis point. We might have been shopping for a bookshelf. Maybe a shower curtain. Whatever it was, I wanted one brand, Ray another.

I turned and walked away. When I was out of sight in another aisle, I started to pace. The splintering. The splintering. My medications weren't working. They couldn't be.

Ray appeared at the end of the aisle looking for me. I pretended to be comparing towel brands. In my hand was an off-white towel, which would have lasted about four seconds with the dust and grime Ray brought home with him from his job.

In the car, he asked what had happened. I couldn't tell him it was from two months of wanting to stay and needing to leave. Two months of holding back the pressure of my *attention deficit disorder/OCD features with some depressive anxious elements*. Two months of trying to be part of a family with all the intimacy and vulnerability and exposure that entailed and at the same time trying to hide. So I said, "I don't know."

That Monday with the sun rising in the city, cloaking the buildings in a cloudy dawn light, I boarded the Megabus. The splintering that had been building all weekend split. Tears. Sobs. In public. Unable to stop.

Ray changed, too. When I met him, he seemed to have gotten over the 2008 financial crisis that had bankrupted him. He was working again after spending nine months collecting unemployment and watching the news, obsessing about the banks being bailed out and executives being offered bonuses. The 2008 crisis had triggered something in him. He'd grown up poor. His father had been bankrupted by the savings and loan crisis of the 1980s and 1990s, when greedy S&L executives defrauded American taxpayers.[1] It had seemed that although the financial crisis had been painful, Ray wasn't consumed by it anymore.

And then he was. He started to listen to audiobooks about it. His voice grew more bitter and menacing with each one. He talked endlessly about the corrupt CEOs and hedge-fund managers, Bernie Madoff, Lehman Brothers, the SEC, laissez-faire free-market economics, former Federal Reserve chairman Alan Greenspan, and Jamie Dimon—he loathed Jamie Dimon.

His paintings became darker. Swirls of thick black and green paint. A fifteen-foot-long canvas of heads piled up, each representing an American who'd been bankrupted.

One night, he stayed up late painting in his studio, drinking wine, and listening to another audiobook about the financial crisis. I'd kissed him good night. He didn't react, so intent was he on the dark painting before him.

I was half-asleep when he came to bed. He said something about Google Maps. Then: "I'm seriously thinking of going to that guy's house and shooting that motherfucker."

I asked who he was talking about.

He named one of the CEOs who'd glided out of the chaos protected by a golden parachute worth millions. Ray had found his address in the Chicago suburbs. "I'm going to kill him," he said.

I believed him. "Ray, you just made me an accomplice. If I don't tell someone—"

"If it weren't for Mikka," he said, his voice hollow, "I'd do it."

The next day, I packed what I needed and left.

Months later, I sat in the hallway of the English-Philosophy Building in Iowa City, waiting to be called into a room to defend my dissertation. Two undergraduate students passed by, the heel of one of their boots squeaking on the linoleum floor. I wasn't nervous, but I should have been.

My breakup with Ray had been swift. The night I left our apartment, I expected to splinter, but I moved back to Iowa full-time into a room in a house with five roommates I barely knew. It was cheap and easy. I focused on finishing my dissertation, which I did in three months.

My thesis advisor came out of the conference room and called me in. I sat at the other end of a long table. On the other side sat my committee: five male professors. I hadn't considered how the dynamics of that would play out.

They questioned me and attacked my dissertation: the argument was weak; the argument didn't carry through; or, as one professor, flustered behind his white beard, put it, he couldn't even find the argument.

I started to shake and fumble my words. A dissertation defense is just that: a defense, which means there's something or someone to defend against. The point was to knock holes in my argument and for me to defend it, but I wasn't prepared. I hadn't asked the other grad students what their defenses had been like. Googling *doctoral defense what like?* never crossed my mind. And my MFA thesis "defense" (though it's hard to call a creative thesis that) had been a veritable lovefest.

Just when I thought I might cry, one of my committee members praised the original research I'd done. Another extolled the writing. They agreed: It was one of the most well-written dissertations they'd ever read. (Not a single comma error in there—I made sure of that.)

Then, somehow, their praise became proof of my dissertation's inadequacy: It was so well written that concentrating on the writing must have distracted me from the argument.

When the defense was over, I sat in the hallway on the same bench and waited for their deliberations to finish. My hands still shook. I eyed the stairwell at the end of the hall and considered walking out and never coming back.

My advisor called me into his office. I stood across from his desk and waited.

"Well," he said, exhaling and sitting down, "you passed."

I asked if it was supposed to be like that.

He shook his head. "They were particularly rough on you. I don't know why."

I left the building and walked out into the chilly fall air. As I headed up the hill on campus, I called my mother and told her. She had a PhD and was overjoyed. When I described how rough it had been, she said, "It doesn't matter. They can never take those three letters away from you."

We ended the call. The splintering sharpened. Classes let out. Students streamed out of buildings and onto the walkway. I hurried away onto the grass as if by bumping into one of them I might break.

———

In my Interpretation of Literature class the following week, a few students had their hands raised to answer the question I'd asked about Toni Morrison's novel *Beloved*. I tried not to praise the literature I taught, letting students have their preferences, but they'd heard me go on about Morrison's novel. It's wrenching and one of the most exquisite novels ever written: gripping plot, finely honed dialogue, richly built characters—though that sounds trite. No summary does it justice, but it centers on a former slave, Sethe, who escapes a plantation only to be found by her "master." (Sethe is based on Margaret Garner, who escaped from slavery in 1856.) To save her children from being recaptured, Sethe tries to kill them, succeeding in killing her oldest, whose tombstone reads *Beloved*.

I asked about Sethe's monologue in the chapter we were reading. We'd gone over how the novel follows African American Vernacular English (AAVE) grammar and punctuation rules. Some of the students thought it was "bad English" or slang, but I explained that AAVE has a distinct set of rules. One mentioned how Sethe says of her daughter "She my daughter" instead of *She's my daughter* and "She mine" instead of *She's mine*. I said it was as if the apostrophe, the possessive, is unnecessary. The student said how that made it seem "like they had this super intense bond."

At the end of class, as the students gathered their things, I put my whiteboard markers in my bag. By the time I got back to my office, the splintering had reached a pitch. But discussing Morrison's novel made me ask what I—someone with freedom and an income and so much privilege—had to be so upset about. Nothing was wrong.

I'm exaggerating. I'm making too big a deal out of nothing.

I might have believed that if I hadn't started crying and dancing in public. The splintering would intensify until it gushed out in tears I couldn't hold back. Sometimes, a high-pitched energy possessed me, and I'd be so revved up and affected by the music I was listening to on my iPod that I danced in the street. After I'd "come down," shame filled me. What if my students had seen? My colleagues? Heavy and unnerved, I pretended it wasn't happening.

———

We like to romanticize, even glamorize, DSM diagnoses: the bipolar artist, the alcoholic writer, the drug-addicted movie star, the schizophrenic genius. A favorite is to anachronistically diagnose artists and writers who were long dead before the diagnoses existed. The Dutch Postimpressionist painter Vincent van Gogh died by suicide and has been posthumously diagnosed with many of the DSM's offerings: bipolar disorder, borderline personality disorder, schizophrenia, schizoaffective disorder, anxiety disorder, and nonsuicidal self-injury disorder.[2] How could he epitomize these different diagnoses, two of which conflict? (Bipolar and schizophrenia are considered mutually exclusive except in the case of schizoaffective disorder, which is a separate diagnosis.)

He can because of two women: Nancy Andreasen and Kay Redfield Jamison. Along with her mental-illness-as-brain-disease proclamations, Andreasen ushered the writer-with-a-mental-illness stereotype into scientific literature. Before becoming a psychiatrist, she was a professor of Renaissance literature (in the same PhD program where I was enrolled—though not at the same time) and was, by her own account, interested in examining how mental illness seemed to be more common in writers and if creativity was genetic.[3] Her 1974 study supposedly proved just that: Writers have a higher rate of mental illness (whether they've been diagnosed or not), it runs in their families, and their family members are more creative, too. Of the *fifteen* "successful creative writers" (what exactly qualifies a writer as "successful" she doesn't say), she wrote, "[T]here *is* [emphasis hers] an association between genius and psychiatric disorder."[4] In the same vein, her 1987 study concluded "there is a close association between mental illness and creativity."[5]

Kay Redfield Jamison, the psychologist and celebrity author, brought Andreasen's theories into the mainstream. (Jamison is often referred to as a psychiatrist, but she has no medical degree.) In 1987, she surveyed forty-seven artists and authors of the British Royal Academy, 38 percent of whom had "been treated" for a mood disorder, which she extrapolated meant they had a mental illness.[6] She helped solidify the public perception of mental illness as "artistic," even sexy, with her subsequent book and memoir. Her 1993 book, *Touched with Fire: Manic-Depressive Illness and the Artistic Temperament,* reinforced the misconception that "crazy" is synonymous with brilliance and artistic genius. Jamison relies primarily on speculation based on biographical information and correspondence. Citing pedigree (genetics), she argues that Lord Byron, Alfred Lord Tennyson, Henry James, Herman Melville, and Vincent van Gogh had manic depression.[7] (It's extremely difficult to imagine Henry James manic.) In *An Unquiet Mind: A Memoir of Moods and Madness*, Jamison shows her struggles with bipolar, but she varnishes them, dramatizing both ends of the bipolar spectrum, so they gleam. Her depressive moods are tragic and her manic experiences are "ecstatic" and "beautifully seductive."[8]

It's tempting to argue that connecting mental illnesses to creativity and genius lessens the stigma. Science journalist Claudia Kalb claims as much in her book, *Andy Warhol Was a Hoarder: Inside the Minds of*

History's Great Personalities, in which she anachronistically diagnoses Albert Einstein with autism and Marilyn Monroe with borderline personality disorder. She writes, "My hope is that telling these stories will highlight the psychological challenges we all face—no matter how big or small—and maybe even eradicate some of the cultural stigma that can go along with them."[9] Andreasen and Jamison may have felt similarly. But a sensationalized view of mental illness could make someone more willing to accept—or embrace—an invalid, unproven DSM diagnosis. If not me, then a teenage girl who has been told by a school psychologist she has ADHD or generalized anxiety disorder or depression or bipolar disorder or all four.

———

On too cold a fall morning to be outside for long, I sat on a bench on the Pedestrian Mall. The cold made my teeth chatter. The outdoor promenade, where students and residents often crowded, was empty of people. Tears streamed down my cheeks. I hovered near hysterics. Then fell into them.

The suicidal thoughts came regularly and then often. The usual: *I can't do this anymore, this is never going to end, I want to die.* They were strongest not at night but midmorning and in the afternoon, often at the campus recreation center after I'd spent an hour on a stair machine or treadmill trying to sweat them away.

I stopped crying long enough to go to my appointment with my therapist, Angela. I'd been seeing her since the depression diagnosis from Dr. B. People said people with depression needed therapy, so I went. The crying, she'd witnessed; the suicidal thoughts, she knew nothing about.

She was young with smiling eyes and a voice that reminded me of a cooing dove. I sat in the client's chair, she opposite me in her desk chair. After some time (therapists like to let you cry), she asked me to talk about it, if I could.

"Nothing's wrong," I said. "That's what I don't understand." I'd passed my dissertation defense. I wasn't sad about Ray anymore.

She asked what else might be causing me to feel the way I did.

The crying started again. It seemed not to come from myself. Then I seemed not to be myself, watching myself in the chair and Angela across from me. I said I didn't want to be there anymore.

Angela clarified: "Where? Here? In the office or . . . ?"

I tried to answer but couldn't. Heaves. Sobs. Ridiculous.

"Have you had these thoughts before?" she asked.

I said I had.

Our session ended. She made me promise to call every day to check in until our next appointment. "I'm responsible for you."

I went to class. I taught. I ran. I wrote. I walked. I ate. I called and checked in.

At my next appointment, Angela asked how I was doing.

"Worse," I said.

She stood and in a gentle voice said she'd be right back. "Don't go anywhere."

I started to cry again.

Angela returned. "We're lucky she's free."

"Who?"

Angela led me down the hall to the office of the psychiatrist in her practice. The psychiatrist's office was painted teal. In her fifties, the psychiatrist had long brown hair and wore a suit jacket, a skirt, and heels. She introduced herself though I can't remember her name.

I sat on the couch. Angela stayed in the room. From the psychiatrist's mouth came questions I tried to answer. I measured my words, modulating my voice so that the words didn't sound alarming. It backfired, and I devolved into hysterics more extreme than if I'd let myself cry.

When I calmed down and looked up, she surprised me: "You don't have ADHD. Or OCD. Or anxiety. Or depression. You're bipolar."

––––––

An exclamation point shouts and in shouting demands attention. By nature, it cries out with emotion. It's a marker of excitability. It also

creates a sense of urgency. It's an interjection (*Wait!*) and an impera-
tive (*Stop!*). It can signify danger.[10]

The prevailing theory is that it was derived from the Latin word
io, meaning an exclamation of joy like *hooray*, in the fifteenth century.[11] Supposedly (though the motivation for this isn't clear), a Roman
started writing the *I* (Romans used all caps) over the *O*; the *O* shrank
by degrees, eventually giving us a line and a dot (*!*). The exclamation
point didn't have its own key on the QWERTY keyboard until 1970.
Prior to that, to exclaim a point required effort. You had to type a period (.), backspace, and then type an apostrophe (*'*.).

It took forty years for the exclamation point to become the hack-
neyed feature of texts and emails. A salutation has to be followed by
one: *Hello!* Simple statements get three, even four: *Can't wait till my
next appointment!!!!* Women are expected to use it more often than
men. It's gendered as a symbol of girlish gushiness.[12]

But it still has the potential to startle, disrupt, and frighten. To indicate extreme pain and fear. To alarm.[13]

———

The psychiatrist smoothed her slacks and stood. "I think you should
see one of my colleagues." She went to the phone on her desk.

"Who?" I asked, panic in my voice.

The psychiatrist didn't answer.

I looked at Angela, whose dove eyes had in them only sympathy.

When the psychiatrist hung up, she said, "We can go."

"Where?" I asked.

She and Angela drove me to a private hospital called Mercy. (The
irony of the name was lost on me at the time.) I was being escorted—
that was clear. An image of my mother and me in the cab on the way to
the eating disorders unit so long ago came to me. I was scared. I wanted
to ask if I'd be able to go home that night. We entered the hospital's
locked, inpatient psychiatric ward. The psychiatrist and Angela led me
to the receptionist.

"Am I being checked in?"

The psychiatrist said, "You'll see someone and decide together."

She and Angela said goodbye. The psychiatrist was all business. Angela looked worried and a little relieved.

I was shown to the day room with the other patients. It had none of the melodrama usually imparted to "psych wards" in movies and in books. The TV on the wall was muted. Four guys sat at a table playing cards. They didn't even look depressed.

On a side table were coffee and tea. The hospital must always be that calm if the staff didn't worry about anyone throwing hot liquid on them or each other, I thought. The room was so quiet that for a moment I wanted to stay.

The room I was assigned had two beds. Panic filled me. "Am I going to have a roommate?" I asked the nurse. It wasn't a hotel moment. I wasn't telling the management the room didn't please me. Sleeping in a room with someone in the same space—with the world so unreal and me disappearing—was impossible. I'd crack for good.

The nurse offered me a benzodiazepine.

"Valium?" I asked.

"Alprazolam." When I didn't respond, she smiled. "Xanax."

"I don't want that. Can I see the doctor?"

After she was gone, I sat on the bed. The thoughts of suicide seemed so irrelevant now that I was being faced with a locked ward. Were they really that serious? They had to be. I was bipolar.

———

The lack of validity of DSM diagnoses and its unstable symptom lists produce statistics that are concerning and absurd. They don't actually tell us the number of Americans with mental disorders; all the statistics really say is that 26 percent or 21 percent (or whatever percentage you want to believe) of American adults receive an invalid, likely unreliable, invented DSM diagnosis (or two) each year.[14]

These statistics are batted about by the media and mental health organizations and on social media as if they're legitimate. Never mind that the diagnoses aren't provable, the statistics don't take the severity of disability into account. The DSM-5 doesn't assess the level of impairment.[15] Depression is depression. Someone with five of nine symptoms has the same diagnosis as someone with all nine. Being a little down is the same as being so depressed as to be suicidal. As others have pointed out, that's like treating a patient with stage 1 cancer the same as one with stage 4 cancer that's metastasized. The DSM only perfunctorily takes the degree and severity of a person's suffering into account.

More compelling statistics come from the NIMH, which at least distinguishes between the rates of any mental illness (AMI) and serious mental illness (SMI).[16] Though some define *serious mental illness* by diagnosis (like bipolar, schizophrenia, and treatment-resistant depression), the NIMH defines it as "serious functional impairment." At least the NIMH's rates of mental illness are more discerning: Although 20 percent of American adults reported any diagnosis (AMI), only 5 percent had a serious mental illness (SMI).[17]

Regardless, the numbers, like the diagnoses, are skewed. How can so many people have DSM diagnoses? The DSM has made it so.

———

The doctor—Dr. C—entered the room. He was young and self-assured. His head was shaved to a pleasant stubble. I remember him being handsome. Something in his face said he wouldn't lie. Maybe it was his confidence or my neediness, the knowledge that I was at risk and only he could save me or set me free.

He sat on the chair across from me and asked questions similar to those the other psychiatrist had asked. When we'd finished, he leaned forward and rested his elbows on his knees. "You have bipolar disorder."

His tone said I should have known, should have been able to identify the highs and lows for what they were: the crying, the dancing. His tone wasn't harsh; in fact, it was supportive. How could I have survived ten or fifteen years without the appropriate treatment? How could I have hidden my illness for that long? How could I have managed my bipolar disorder without help?

My bipolar disorder.

———

Bipolar is all about extremes. The bipolar patient shifts between two states: depression and mania. In mania, she's been described as fitting one of two subtypes: euphoric-grandiose or paranoid-destructive.[18] In depression, she's simply depressed.

Bipolar has been identified by different names and as having different causes, all of which have been grim. Hippocrates and the ancient Greeks identified it as the fluctuation between an excess of black and yellow bile.[19] It had the distinct pleasure of being referred to as "circular insanity" by the French psychiatrist Jean-Pierre Falret in 1851. Kraepelin called it "manic-depressive insanity" in 1899, grouping all mood states (depressive, manic, and mixed) on a spectrum.[20]

Our modern concept of the illness didn't start until 1966, when Jules Angst, a Swiss psychiatrist, and Carlo Perris, a Swedish psychiatrist, distinguished unipolar depression (just depression) from bipolar depression (depression with mania). But the distinction made between unipolar and bipolar depression and the many subtypes and categories invented over the half century that followed didn't make bipolar a scientifically reliable diagnosis. Unipolar and bipolar depression can look alike, especially in someone who's high energy (e.g., me). It can be hard to tell if a patient is experiencing an extremely low mood with some days or weeks of reprieve (unipolar depression) or low mood with days or weeks of manic highs (bipolar disorder).

The DSM's definition of *bipolar* changed over the five editions.[21] The DSM-I considered *manic-depressive reaction*, as it was called, a psychotic condition with a psychological cause, not a physical one. Marked by severe mood swings, it could also include delusions and hallucinations. The DSM-II renamed it *manic-depressive illness*, characterizing it in terms of mood shifts unrelated to life events: manic, depressed, and "circular." Manic type presented with elation, irritability, talkativeness, and increased activity with few bouts of depression. Depressed type resembled what I experienced: extremely low mood, apprehension, and agitation. "Circular" meant a mix of manic and depressive symptoms.

The DSM-III renamed it *bipolar disorder* and created more rigid categories for what constituted a manic, a depressive, or a mixed episode. The DSM-IV invented a brand-new unproven diagnosis: bipolar II. In the DSM-5, bipolar disorder was given its own category, no longer binned among other mood and affective disorders, creating a "bipolar spectrum."[22]

Depressive symptoms I had in spades: low energy, agitation, a sense of worthlessness, loss of interest in life (except for teaching, yes), insomnia, suicidality. Mine had come on fast and without cause—a hallmark of bipolar.

But had I been manic? For signs of mania, the psychiatrist and Dr. C would have found few: distractible (that word again), hyperactive (a little—is that possible?), markedly energetic (perhaps), experiencing flights of ideas (yes), feeling as though I didn't need sleep (I wasn't sleeping, but need was a separate issue).

That didn't seem to matter. The psychiatrist and Dr. C saw in me someone with bipolar disorder. I could either become it or not.

———

Sitting across from Dr. C, I listened to the wind outside. Tree branches knocked against the window. *Bipolar.* I wanted out.

"Please," I said, "don't make me stay here."

He eyed me and asked if I thought I was a danger to myself.

I shook my head. "I'm fine."

He leaned back in his chair. "Given the thoughts you've been having . . . but I can't keep you here." I didn't have a plan, no clear way to end my life.

"The thoughts are gone."

"For now," he said.

"I'll be fine."

He looked at me sidelong. "What will you do?"

"Laundry," I said. Never had I wanted to do laundry so much—something methodical, predictable, real.

"That's a good sign," he said and smiled.

I walked down Bloomington Street, trying to understand how the psychiatrist and Dr. C had made the leap from ADHD and OCD and depression and anxiety to bipolar disorder. If two psychiatrists had said it, it must be true. That meant my primary care physician had been wrong. For years. And years.

When I got home, one of my roommates, a German undergraduate student, was in the kitchen. Her long hair hung down almost to her waist. She smiled and held aloft a pint of Häagen-Dazs vanilla ice cream. Did I want a bowl?

It was such a simple question, such an ordinary action: eat a bowl of ice cream. I'd just been in a locked ward because I'd considered ending my life. How to reconcile that alongside her scooping sweet vanilla ice cream into a bowl? I thanked her and shook my head.

In my room, I did what anyone would do: I googled. The internet was a font of confirmation. There were options: I could be bipolar I or bipolar II. Random searches told me that 60 percent of people with bipolar disorder are misdiagnosed, some of them for more than ten years.[23] (That sounded like me.) Though the age of onset of bipolar disorder in women was typically twenties and thirties, being diagnosed in one's forties was common enough. (I was close.)

I started to see the symptoms in myself. Mania meant increased activity (maybe), less need for sleep (I was a grad student—that was my special skill), overly euphoric or irritable mood (sure, both), risky or impulsive behaviors (I'd had sex with someone I barely knew), racing thoughts (in spades), rapid speech (maybe).[24] Depression meant sadness, anxiety, feelings of guilt and worthlessness, loss of interest in life, difficulty sleeping, suicidal thoughts (yes, yes, yes, yes, yes, and yes).[25] External factors weren't to blame. I didn't use substances, which meant it couldn't be a substance abuse disorder.

The idea of rejecting my diagnosis never crossed my mind. But I didn't say to myself that the psychiatrist and Dr. C could be wrong either; I just put aside their words—*my bipolar*—and didn't repeat them, not even when seated across from Angela at our next session, light streaming in from the window.

10

When the Happy Pill Ends

The office of my new therapist, Amy, was on the seventeenth floor of an office building not far from the Art Institute of Chicago. Her chair was close to mine—a couple feet away—and she rested her clogs on a tiny stool. She didn't cover the gray in her hair and wore no visible makeup. She pronounced *human* without the *h* ("you're *yuman*," she'd say), which was more distracting than it should have been. I'd found her on the internet.

We talked a lot about relationships. Her favorite metaphor was that of a puzzle with many pieces, each of the pieces a person in one's life. "You get to decide who goes in the center and who belongs on the outer edges."

I didn't ask what that meant to someone who had a puzzle with few pieces. In Iowa, the crying had eased up and the suicidal thoughts had faded by the time I received my doctorate. My move back to Chicago had been motivated by the need to be somewhere solid, familiar—home. I was staying with my mother—until I found a place. I taught adjunct at two universities. Teaching constituted the majority of my social life. This didn't bother me. Solitaries like small puzzles. Mine didn't need many pieces.

As with Anne and Angela, with Amy, I tended to complain a lot—pointless indulgent complaining. Amy always agreed with me, which I both liked and didn't. The result was often conspiratorial, the two of us judging my family and others in ways that seemed unfair.

My mother knew about the suicidal thoughts and the hospital. Our relationship changed. The presumption now was that I was fragile. I'd been suicidal.

Neither she nor Amy knew about the bipolar diagnosis. I couldn't pretend the months of crying and the suicidal thoughts and the hospital hadn't happened, but I wasn't ready. It was obviously more than *attention deficit disorder/OCD features with some depressive anxious elements*. And my logic was starting to become circular. If I had a mental illness and it wasn't *attention deficit disorder/OCD features with some depressive anxious elements*, it had to be something else because I'd been diagnosed, which meant I had to have a diagnosis.

Dr. H was my first real psychiatrist. In his tiny waiting room, classical music played from a small speaker on the side table. Next to it were copies of *TIME*. He opened the door and invited me in. I sat in a stiff armchair at one end of the room and he in an Eames Lounge Chair positioned on the other. He had reddish hair and was slight of frame.

He asked me questions about my diagnoses and my medications. I told him about the hospital and the psychiatrist and Dr. C. I had to tell him. What if I became suicidal again?

At the end of our session, he nodded and squinched his nose as if smelling something bad. Then he said I may not have ADHD. Or OCD. Or depression. Or anxiety. I might be bipolar.

"I just don't see myself as bipolar," I said.

He said, "No, I would put you in the category of bipolar II."

I passed through the revolving doors of his office building. It was still tentative: *May not have ADHD or OCD or depression or anxiety. May/may not. May*—that modal verb that provided escape, not certainty.

In the almost-twilight, I crossed the street on Dearborn. Cars stopped at the crosswalk to let people pass. The Ritalin wasn't helping (was it?) and the SSRI was (wasn't it?). But three psychiatrists couldn't be wrong.

The internet offered many convincing reasons to believe the psychiatrist and Dr. C and Dr. H were right. I only needed to have had one major depressive episode in my lifetime (check) and one hypomanic episode. Manic didn't sound like me, but hypomania seemed like manic lite. And didn't I sometimes have inflated self-esteem (I'd thought my committee would see only good in my dissertation), feel rested after around three hours of sleep (check), exhibit risky behavior with money (I'd also blown my savings to rehab a loft not zoned for residential), and have racing thoughts (double check)? Couldn't I be more talkative than usual (I was known to talk fast), distractible (I'd been ADHD seconds before), and overly goal directed (only always)?

Hypomania wasn't just euphoria and grandiosity; it was characterized by agitation and "persistently elevated" irritability, too. And weren't those terrible surges of energy agitation? And didn't I go dark for days at a time? Not depression dark; closed-off, don't-come-near-me dark, a kind of force field that signaled to my mother to stay away. I'd be in the kitchen making my lunch for teaching the next day at one of the universities where I taught. When my mother would come in, I'd stiffen. The dark irritability force field would fill the space around me. I didn't want to be that way. After she walked out, I wanted to call after her and apologize, but it was like being trapped.

WebMD and Healthline said bipolar II was a lesser version of bipolar I.[1] Verywell Mind told me I could function okay with it, which maybe I'd been able to, for the most part, never having to cancel a class, never missing a deadline.[2]

Suicidality—a term I learned and started to use with frequency— was more likely in people with bipolar than in those with depression.[3] And what if it returned? With a different diagnosis and different medications, couldn't I ensure it wouldn't?

When I told my mother I was bipolar II, she looked worried. Then she said, "Okay, we'll do whatever we need to do."

———

My diagnosis occurred during another DSM-driven "epidemic": bipolar II.[4] The epidemic occurred, in part, because the DSM-IV relied on the defining symptom of hypomania instead of mania. In bipolar II, hypomania is defined as four days of persistently elevated, expansive, or irritable mood with at least three of the following (or four, if the mood was only irritability): grandiosity, decreased need for sleep, talkativeness, racing thoughts, distractibility, increased goal-directed activity or psychomotor agitation, or excessive involvement in pleasurable and risky behaviors. Researchers later found that the DSM's definition of hypomania isn't scientifically valid.[5] Anyone can be grandiose at times. How decreased does the need for sleep have to be? Is talkativeness really a symptom? Technically, we all have racing thoughts and are distractible. Don't we praise those who are goal-oriented, particularly those who are intensely so? Doesn't the media urge us to seek out pleasurable activities, even those that might be risky?

Allen Frances defended the DSM-IV's broadening criteria by saying it was done to prevent patients from being diagnosed with depression, put on an antidepressant, and having a manic episode.[6] Taking Frances's and the DSM's cue, others wanted to add yet more subtypes. Psychiatrist and researcher David Dunner argued in favor of a bipolar spectrum that included not only bipolar II, but also bipolar III.[7] The psychiatrist Hagop Akiskal claimed the existence of bipolar IV.[8] Others have said it should include "sporadic brief hypomania" during which symptoms need only last for at least one day and occur no more than once a month.[9]

It came down to words on a page. The DSM-IV's definition made it hard to distinguish between a hypomanic high and a regular old good mood that lasts four days. Although it did specify that hypomania "is clearly different from the usual nondepressed mood," the criteria didn't specify what the difference between an episode and a "usual nondepressed mood" might be.[10] After all, someone in a really good mood—or even just a good mood—might feel "a decreased need for sleep," be more involved in "goal-directed activity," and pursue "pleasurable activities" that involve risk.

In the two decades following the publication of the DSM-IV, some urged restraint and questioned bipolar's clinical popularity, but it was too late.[11] Drug companies seized the opportunity, advertising to consumers that any elevation in mood or irritability mixed with low mood was a sign they—we—were bipolar. The result was overdiagnosis.[12]

Allen Frances later (too late) regretted the words that made bipolar II so easy to diagnose, but it took him fifteen years to speak out. Only then did he blog, tweet, and publish articles and a book to both admit to and deny wrongdoing.[13]

In *Saving Normal*, he doesn't exactly offer a mea culpa; he still shirks the blame, pointing the finger at drug companies (whose purpose on this planet, as we all know and they don't deny, is to make money by getting people to take their drugs). He acknowledges the DSM-IV's role in creating the false epidemics of bipolar II, autism, and ADHD.[14] The DSM-IV could have prevented those "epidemics" by requiring more symptoms of longer duration with greater impairment.

His apologies are qualified with *probably*. The DSM-IV "probably" did more harm than good[15] and could have and "probably" should have worked toward diagnostic deflation.[16] The authors could have warned the American public of the risk of overdiagnosis[17] and should have thought about how clinicians and others would implement the manual they'd written and should have acknowledged that 56 percent of the "experts" who worked on the DSM-IV had financial ties to drug companies.[18] But still, Frances writes, it wouldn't have mattered; they "probably couldn't have stemmed the tide of overdiagnosis," as if he could possibly know.[19]

He blames psychiatrists who treated the DSM, psychiatry's bible, as if it were the Bible. The DSM-IV, he writes, wasn't a catalog of "'real' diseases," just "useful diagnostic constructs." After all, the coauthors stated as much in the introduction.[20] But Frances writes that he wasn't sure "anyone ever reads" the introduction and "few people have read" (really read) the DSM's Guidebook, which qualifies DSM diagnoses.[21]

He portrays himself as naive, someone who never could have guessed that the DSM-IV's loose diagnostic criteria would allow drug companies to exploit diagnoses like bipolar II.[22] He writes this while at the same time admitting he'd witnessed how the DSM-III-R caused the Prozac boom: "Prozac and DSM-III-R were both introduced in 1987. Prozac's sales took off at least in part because the DSM definition of major depressive disorder was so loose. The message was clear— psychotropic drugs offered vast market potential, and sales could be greatly influenced by DSM decisions."[23]

Frances chalks up the damage caused by the DSM-IV to "silly mistakes"[24] necessary to fill "an important clinical niche." None of it's a very big deal. He writes, "We didn't do much harm, but we weren't of much help."

Didn't do much harm.

———

The first line of treatment was to change my medications. Dr. H took me off Ritalin, which, he said, was the worst medication someone with bipolar could be on. The week after I was off it, he said I'd stay on the SSRI. We'd add a mood stabilizer, lamotrigine (an anticonvulsant used to treat epilepsy that moonlighted as a mood stabilizer), the side effects of which included Stevens-Johnson syndrome, a reddish-purple rash that could "eat" my flesh and possibly kill me. He assured me it was rare.

After six months of teaching and writing and being on lamotrigine, no flesh-eating rash had appeared. Dr. H asked how I was feeling on it.

"Fine," I said, "but not that different."

A squinch. A nod. "Good. That means it's working."

———

It wasn't. After months of splintering and cracking and decidedly unstable moods (despite the mood stabilizer), I started to have panic attacks. They were unlike any I'd ever known: deep, suffocating, vertigo inducing. The four together—splintering, cracking, mood swings, and panic attacks—soon brought thoughts of suicide.

Dr. H and I made an emergency plan. If my suicidal thoughts returned, I should go to Northwestern's inpatient psychiatric unit. (This wasn't the same eating disorders unit where I'd been an outpatient as an anorexic. Northwestern's eating disorders unit had long since closed, its circular building demolished. Only the most severe eating disorder cases were treated inpatient.) I asked what would happen if I went. He said its admission process was separate from the emergency room's. I'd go right in.

That was the day my mother and I wandered around in the heat looking for a nonexistent separate entrance to the inpatient psych unit. I called Dr. H several times. He didn't call back. The longer we looked, the more worried my mother became.

By the time we were inside the emergency room and my name had been called and the nurse had taken my blood pressure and listened to my heart and told us the psychiatric unit was a closed ward and there was no telling what hospital I'd end up in, Dr. H still hadn't called back.

When my mother and I got home, she sat on the couch and I on the chair across from her. She asked how Dr. H could have been so wrong. I said I didn't know.

Eventually, my cell phone rang. I told Dr. H there hadn't been a separate admissions procedure and likely the psych unit wouldn't have had any beds available. Nonplussed, he said it wasn't like that before. I could almost feel him shrug, *Oh, well.* He didn't apologize, just told me he hadn't had to "deal" with a suicidal patient in a long time.

————

I was a particular kind of suicidal. Not suicidal like those facing end-of-life or death-with-dignity decisions. Not as someone trying to make a religious or political statement. It would have been described as "despair"[25] suicidality in the sense of "deaths of despair,"[26] a term coined by Anne Case and Angus Deaton at Princeton University to describe premature mortality involving drugs, alcohol, or suicide.[27] That kind of despair—giving up, being unable to see the possibility of a positive future—can be cognitive (pessimism, worthlessness, helplessness), emotional (apathy, sadness, irritability), behavioral (self-destructive acts, recklessness, inaction), and biological (stress-related illnesses).

For me, it was the result of too many days of a hopelessness so pene-
trating it hollowed me out.

———

I didn't trust Dr. H anymore. It wasn't so much the inadequacy of his
emergency plan; it was his ambivalence. If I was that sick, I needed the
right care.

After googling for some time, I found a "bipolar specialist." It
seemed too good to be true: an expert in my particular illness, my diagnosis, my bipolar. Dr. M would be all to me: psychiatrist and therapist.

The waiting room of his office offered filtered water and little Dixie
cups. On the phone, he'd said we'd meet to determine if we were "the
right fit." I'd already talked myself into believing that he—the bipolar
expert—would help me make sense of my life, my thoughts, my diagnosis, my mind, once and for all.

The door opened. A blond, bright but serious man poked his head
out and called me in. He wore a comfy-looking cardigan sweater. His
blond hair was stiff and well coiffed. He was young but gave off an air
of quiet confidence.

I stood and followed him down a hallway of closed office doors
behind which were the other psychiatrists in his practice.

His office was windowless and small. I sat on the gray couch—fake
leather and overly cushioned. He sat in a desk chair close by.

On his desk behind him was a can of grapefruit LaCroix. It read,
Naturally Essenced Sparkling Water. Essenced seemed to come from a
place where water sparkled and nothing ever went wrong.

For forty minutes, he asked me about my mental health history
and a bit about my life. I told him about the other diagnoses and the
hospital in Iowa and the image of me in the bathtub in Chicago—all
of it. When we finished, I asked if I was bipolar. He was the expert. He
would know.

Turning to his desk, he picked up the LaCroix can. I wondered if
he'd mind that it was warm. He faced me again, can in hand.

Yes, I was bipolar—bipolar II. He slipped his finger under the tab and opened the can. When the scent of grapefruit reached me, it tasted of relief.

That night, I filled out the "life chart" Dr. M assigned me. Seated at the desk in my mother's study, I colored in the graph provided, blocking out years and writing in events, shading the highs and lows that could be considered bipolar episodes. It had the look of real data, bars jutting above the zero axis—the "normal" axis—and others falling below it: months when the black mass or the sodden pit was there and my mind slowed; days and weeks when the splintering and cracking happened and I'd felt an urgent need to run or walk or dance to music only I could hear; the grandiose plans I'd had to finish my dissertation in three months (which I did) and still had to finish a novel in about the same amount of time (which I didn't). My life was no longer divided into weeks and months and years; it was made up of manic and depressive episodes.

I leaned back in my chair and stared down at the chart. Twenty years of hypomanic highs and depressive lows, twenty years of undiagnosed bipolar disorder. I put down my pen.

———

My sessions with Dr. M revolved around my illness. His questions reframed events and interactions in terms of *my bipolar*. My past became reordered. Memories played at a slower or faster speed. The motivations behind this or that decision were different now that I saw them through the lens of bipolarity.

He was the Sherman to my Kessa. His presence—just his presence— promised I'd never be suicidal again. The time between our sessions was interminable. Always there loomed the threat of another episode— depressive or manic—worse than the one before. Only he had the answer.

With him, I managed my new life as someone with bipolar. *Managed* was a word I heard and read a lot. Manage, meaning *handle*. Manage, meaning *cope*.

I learned more about bipolar disorder than any layperson should know. I subscribed to *BP Hope*, a magazine for people with bipolar.

The *My Story* column featured people who revealed their long battles with bipolar disorder—a country musician, an ex-model, a lawyer. I turned page after page of drug ads for Latuda and Abilify and other antipsychotics to the *Ask the Doctor* column, which covered the many medications I had to choose from.

My mother asked to read it because she wanted to learn how to better support me. I let her. When she finished and handed me the magazine, her face was clouded with concern. "Are you sure you want to read that?"

I said, "Of course," and asked why.

"It's just so . . . dark."

The internet offered so much information—so much contradictory information—about the natural remedies I could add. Folic acid and vitamin B12 were crucial to sound mental health; no, magnesium was.[28] A high-fat, low-carb diet caused depression; no, a low-fat, high-carb diet did. Green and black teas were high in the amino acid L-theanine, which relieved stress and anxiety but caffeine triggered manic episodes. The Mediterranean diet was the key to relieving depression but particularly in smokers.[29] Blogs on the Harvard Health website reported that there was "overwhelming evidence" for a connection between food and mental health though others insisted further studies were urgently required to elucidate whether a "true causal association exists."[30] I scrolled down the *Medical News Today* website, past an ad for Vraylar, an antipsychotic as yet unknown to me, to be told once again that bipolar might be caused by a chemical imbalance that may or may not be helped by fish oil and vitamin C.[31]

Website after website confirmed that my prognosis was grave. With the diagnosis, my life expectancy had shortened by nine to twenty years.[32] The illness would worsen over time, each manic or depressive occurrence increasing that likelihood.[33] With each depressive episode, my risk of having dementia rose.[34] There was a very good chance I'd never have a long-term relationship or hold a regular job. I'd relapse. I'd end my own life.

The inevitable was coming: early death, more frequent episodes, relapses, suicide. I admitted to myself that I was, in fact, living—not staying—with my mother. I registered with a disability at one of the universities where I worked. My diet was impeccable, my sleep regular (when I wasn't in an episode), and my schedule precise. I rarely went out at night—or during the day, except to teach, walk, and run. I wrote my novel. I read. I watched Netflix. I prepped classes. I taught.

I lost count of the number of times Dr. M told me how ill I was. The premise of our work together was that I was very, very sick. Occasionally, he agreed—with person-first consideration—that I was someone *with* a mental illness, not "mentally ill." I was, as the cliché goes, "more than my illness."

It's not as if I could have questioned my diagnosis. Not admitting I was bipolar indicated a "lack of insight," anosognosia, which meant I was in denial, which meant I was sicker than I thought.

———

Four months later, Dr. M said it was time to stop the SSRI.

"Really?" I asked.

He said that antidepressants could induce mania in bipolar patients and long-term use could spur more episodes and potentially cause something called *rapid cycling*, a pattern of moving more quickly between periods of depression and mania.

I thought of how I'd stood at my kitchen counter five years earlier with the SSRI—that orange, oblong pill—between my fingers. How nimbly I'd swallowed it. Within minutes (seconds?), my mind had stilled, and I'd entered a sea of calm. Innocuous. Palatable. A simple adjustment.

"It's helped," I said.

He shook his head. "It won't for long." The literature, a term he used often to assert his authority, agreed he was right.

———

Later I'd learn that "the literature" didn't fully support his conclusion.[35] Until 2002, antidepressants were used as the first line of treatment in bipolar disorder and although some of the older antidepressants seemed to trigger manic episodes, similar evidence with modern antidepressants—like SSRIs—was lacking.[36] According to studies, the risk of my illness worsening as a result of the SSRI was 12 percent; the likelihood of improvement was 41 percent.[37]

If I'd known that becoming bipolar would mean going off my SSRI and that going off my SSRI would lead to eight months of severe withdrawal symptoms, I might never have let that oblong orange pill slide down my throat. Dr. B didn't mention that if, after five years, I tried to go off it, it wouldn't be a simple adjustment, nothing like taking off a pair of glasses.

In some ways, it wasn't Dr. B's fault—not really. If a certain 1996 symposium had never taken place, I might never have ended up in those emergency rooms and partial hospitalization programs. In Phoenix, Arizona, seven psychiatrists—Alan Schatzberg, Eric Kaplan, Peter Haddad, Michel Lejoyeux, Allan Young, Jerrold Rosenbaum, and John Zajecka—gathered at the behest (and expense) of Eli Lilly, maker of the SSRI Prozac, before releasing a report that denied SSRIs can have withdrawal symptoms as severe as some narcotics. Pharmaceutical companies had been aware of people suffering symptoms like mine— brain zaps, involuntary muscle twitching, paranoia, nightmares, crying spells—for almost thirty years and still pretended it wasn't true.[38] In a report and editorials and papers published after the symposium, they named it *SSRI discontinuation syndrome* because SSRIs weren't associated with dependence and took too long to work. They insisted SSRI discontinuation syndrome (some called it *SRI discontinuation syndrome*—"serotonin reuptake inhibitor" without *selective*) was "generally mild and transient, and . . . self-limiting," based on no clinical data. Symptoms were merely "troublesome" and could "lead to missed work days."[39] Nothing more.

Without Eli Lilly and those seven "key opinion leaders," as pharmaceutical companies call doctors whose research they fund, Dr. B might have known to warn me that going off my SSRI—my supposed "happy pill," which never made me smiley-face happy but did slow my racing thoughts—would lead to eight months of anxiety and paranoia, akathisia and confusion, sweating and agitation, insomnia and nightmares, and crying spells and seeing things and people who weren't there.

And brain shivers, which made me feel like a waterfall of needles was cascading down the back of my head.

And brain shudders, which felt like my mind was trembling.

And brain zaps, which made me feel like I was being electrocuted.

———

Two months into my withdrawal—two months of tapering, each subtraction of a milligram of my SSRI another zap or shiver or bout of confusion—I sat beside my mother on her blue couch. Staring down at my feet, I traced the pattern of her Oriental rug so as not to look at my shaking hands. She sat beside me, her brow furrowed again. I tried to explain what was happening with the withdrawal. But telling her about the brain shivers and brain zaps and seeing things that weren't there would have upset her too much. So I told her about the trembling and sweating and crying spells and rushes of panic.

She said I should call Dr. M. Even I could hear the panic in my voice as I left him a message.

We waited. My mother rubbed my back the way she had when I was a child. In time to the arcs drawn by the movement of her fingers, I traced the curves in the design of her blue carpet.

Dr. M called back at ten minutes to the hour. He must have listened to my message right after his previous patient left.

"My brain feels foggy," I said after I'd told him a short, sanitized version of what was happening. His voice was concerned, steady. As he spoke—reassuring, planning what to do next—I told myself I'd be fine. Everything would be fine.

———

Trust is more of a transaction than an emotion. There are two parties: the trustor and the trustee. The transaction will take place in the future.

By placing herself in the trustee's hands and at his whims, the trustor has no power.

When the word came into English in the Middle Ages, it had more to do with religious faith than relying on someone with power and having that trust honored. But it wasn't long before it became tied up in the honesty of the person trusted.

The psychologist Erik Erikson said trust is the first stage of psychosocial development, lasting from birth until around eighteen months. If children learn they can trust their caregiver, they'll be able to form trusting relationships and secure attachments throughout their life. If they learn they can't, they're more likely to go through life with anxious attachment, insecurity, and fear.

As adults, trust prevents us from getting stuck in "analysis paralysis." It allows us to move forward and past the boundaries set by our rational minds. One could argue trust is delusional. It's privileging a delusion (the trustee's reliability and honesty, which may or may not be there) over reality (the inability to know for sure).

———

Four months into my withdrawal, I sat in my windowless office at the university where I taught, trying to prep for class. It was a Tuesday. It was April. The papers on my desk seemed far away though they were right in front of me. My pen was pressed to one of them. I forgot what I was going to write, something about the text we were reading, something about—

An electric zap shot through my brain. I closed my eyes and leaned forward, resting my head in my hands. It was startling, the power of the zap, how it reverberated.

My instinct was to push through the zaps and shudders and shivers. As I reached for my notes for class, my hand shook. I stood, unsteady. More than unsteady. Like I didn't have legs. They were disconnected as if they didn't belong to my body or to me.

I left my office, having to return twice when I realized that I'd forgotten my water bottle and my copy of the text. With my bag slumped over my shoulder, I made my way through the sea of students in the hallway. It was a sea, my body a buoy bobbing among them.

Midway down the hall, I strengthened. Being in motion helped. My legs woke. Except I wasn't convinced I was real. The bag on my shoulder might have been on someone else's shoulder. Me but not me. My shoulder but not my shoulder.

The students who'd arrived early sat in their now-familiar seats. Most stared down at their cell phones. A few tapped their screens. Others scrolled and scrolled.

At the front of the room, I stood behind the podium and logged on to the computer. On-screen, the home page of the course website quivered as if there were about to be an outage. I looked away.

Two students whooshed in the door, talking animatedly. Their voices were loud and tinny. They sat in the back row, still talking. One said something about a parking violation. Or an accident? Their voices faded in and out.

I wrote the date on the whiteboard. The glare of the fluorescent lights was too bright. I stopped writing and looked down at the speckled brown carpeting.

The thought of canceling class didn't cross my mind. It was something I didn't do. My professional standard.

I took attendance and stood at the front of the room, not having finished what I was writing on the board. Half the date was up there, written in black marker, alone with nothing after it, as if the time we spent in class would never end and existed in a void.

My legs became shaky again. I leaned on the podium to steady myself.

We delved into a discussion about (ironically) a piece of long-form journalism by Gabriel Mac (née Mac McClelland) about the failure of the mental health system. My students liked talking about mental health, which they referred to as mental illness. Given how many of them had come to my office hours to share that they suffered from ADHD or anxiety or depression or were bipolar, I assumed that was why. They were a pathologized generation, used to being told that distraction meant ADHD, sadness meant depression, and worry meant an anxiety disorder. Few were registered with the Center for Students with Disabilities. There could have been a million reasons for this—stigma being the big one—but it sometimes made me skeptical. They were so used to seeing mental illness portrayed dramatically and hyperbolically in YA novels and on TV shows and in movies. Why wouldn't they think everyone had it? Why wouldn't their adolescent minds tap into it as an explanation? But a part of me wanted to say, *Of course you have anxiety. You're in college. You're given quizzes and forced to take tests and are graded. That's anxiety inducing.* Other times, I believed every one of them had the mental illness they'd been diagnosed with. Did they already refer to their "ADHD brains"? Had they already been put on SSRIs to manage their anxiety or depression? How many of them had been told it would be a simple adjustment, just like wearing glasses?

I asked about the author's use of form in the piece, how it moved in and out of personal experience and facts about the mental health system. One student—one of the boisterous ones in the back—informed us that that part was "boring."

I asked more questions. Some of the students picked up the thread of the discussion and sewed it among themselves.

When that trailed off, I asked another question. One of the students—always attentive—started to answer. In my vision, she started to blur or, rather, cloud over. It was as if I'd stood too quickly and the room was fading, except I was still leaning on the desk.

I somehow got through the ninety-minute class. Afterward, without stopping at my office, I went outside. It was a bright, early spring afternoon, unseasonably warm, enough not to wear a coat. I was shaking.

I called Dr. M. He didn't answer. I left a message and paced.

When he returned my call, I had already decided to take myself to the emergency room. Something was very wrong, I told him. He reminded me that I was coming off the SSRI. I told him about the worsening brain zaps and not being able to hear what my students were saying and the cloudiness. He reminded me that "could" happen when discontinuing an SSRI.

We hung up. I wobbled and leaned on a small city tree to steady myself. Dragging my fingers along its rough bark, I told myself I'd be off the SSRI soon. Then I remembered Dr. M had said the last milligrams were the worst.

———

When I started my SSRI, the chemical imbalance theory of mental illness had already been debunked, but—thanks to psychiatry's failure to be forthcoming, big pharma's stake in the theory, and the media's weakness for repeating false claims—it remained a publicly sanctioned cultural myth.[40] The chemical imbalance theory says that mental illnesses like depression are supposedly caused by a deficit of neurotransmitters like norepinephrine, dopamine, and serotonin. Many biological psychiatrists promise that one day (someday, even though it hasn't happened in thirty years of research) it will be proven true; regardless, it wasn't true when I took that first orange oblong pill and it isn't true today. There are an unknown number of neurotransmitters in the brain, and researchers don't know how they work.

When it was first hypothesized by the psychiatrist Joseph Schildkraut in 1965, the chemical imbalance theory was little more than conjecture.[41] Schildkraut himself doubted his idea that depression was caused by norepinephrine (not serotonin, which is how it's described today) but thought *maybe* it *could* be. It isn't.

Yet the chemical imbalance theory hung around, perhaps because it's convenient to pharmaceutical companies and biological psychiatrists, who want us to think that DSM diagnoses are biological. Their thinking goes something like this: DSM diagnoses haven't been shown to be caused by a chemical imbalance in the brain but pharmaceutical drugs affect neurotransmitters and are prescribed to treat DSM diagnoses, so DSM diagnoses must be caused by a chemical imbalance. As with Dr. B and his belief that I had ADHD because Ritalin "seemed to be working," the drugs are said to prove not only the unproven diagnosis but also its unproven cause.

Even that isn't true. In 1998, psychotherapist and researcher Irving

Kirsch published a meta-analysis "Listening to Prozac but Hearing Placebo" which found that antidepressants were only effective 25 percent of the time.[42] Another 25 percent was due to "nonspecific factors" and 50 percent to the placebo effect. (Kirsch wasn't actually interested in antidepressants; his research was on the placebo effect: how the hope or belief in an inactive pill can create the same healing effect as an active one.) Kirsch was criticized for handpicking studies that would prove his point, but he did a second analysis that demonstrated the same results.[43] He also wasn't alone. Other researchers conducted studies on antidepressants and the placebo effect that echoed Kirsch's findings.[44]

His follow-up book *The Emperor's New Drugs: Exploding the Antidepressant Myth* gave him fifteen seconds of fame. Kirsch and his book were featured in *Newsweek* and a segment about him aired on *60 Minutes*. In a review published in the *New York Review of Books*, Marcia Angell, one-time editor of the influential *New England Journal of Medicine*, heaped praise on the book.[45]

But the repudiation of the chemical imbalance myth didn't catch on. And why would it have? In direct-to-consumer advertisements, drug companies like Eli Lilly and Pfizer advertised that SSRIs like Prozac and my very own Zoloft promised to raise serotonin levels and ease depression. The result was billions of dollars in revenue for Eli Lilly and Pfizer and others and people who believed that if they received a DSM diagnosis and a prescription, they must have a chemical imbalance. The media played its part.[46] As early as the 1970s, articles about it had appeared in the *New York Times* and *Cosmopolitan*.[47] Even today, websites like Healthline cloud the facts *by kind of* telling people that the chemical imbalance theory is false but then running headlines that declare it's what they'll be treated for.[48]

Ronald Pies, a clinical professor of psychiatry, defends psychiatry's role in proselytizing the chemical imbalance theory. He admits it's an "urban myth" and little more than an effect of psychiatry's "high school crush" on serotonin, but it's okay that it's an urban myth and it's not true and we've been led to believe that it is.[49] Pies says, yes, plenty of psychiatrists use the term *chemical imbalance* when handing a patient a DSM diagnosis. He then argues that no, psychiatry isn't to blame because, after all, *some* psychiatrists *don't* talk about the chemical imbalance theory.[50]

That's the problem. Mental health professionals don't say to their patients, *Oh, by the way, that whole chemical-imbalance theory we talked about all those years and staked our reputations on and continued to let you believe isn't true.* How likely would a patient be to adopt a diagnosis if a doctor said, *Well, you may have clinical depression, but we don't know what causes it and it's certainly not caused by a chemical imbalance in the brain and, in fact, we can't scientifically validate what depression actually is but here, take this prescription for a drug that may work—though we don't really know how—and which may have terrible side effects and which you may have to continue taking because the withdrawal can be vicious*?

Some argue that, well, it's okay to make people think the chemical imbalance theory is true because it gives us an answer to the causes of our suffering that makes it easier for us to accept DSM diagnoses without seeing ourselves as flawed. And doesn't it reduce stigma? No, actually, it doesn't. One study showed that attaching a supposed biological cause to a diagnosis produces *more* shame, pessimism, negativity, and hopelessness about the future.[51]

Of course, the DSM never said—outright—that I or anyone else had or has a chemical imbalance, but it said my diagnosis might be biological, so what was I to think? Didn't Nancy Andreasen declare, "These diseases [DSM diagnoses] are caused principally by biological factors"?[52] Didn't medical textbooks and others say the same?[53] Didn't the DSMs III, III-R, IV, IV-TR, and 5 state—in writing—that their diagnoses might have a biological component? Wasn't a chemical imbalance in the brain biological?

The DSM didn't make me swallow that orange oblong pill. Psychiatry's bible actually offers no treatment suggestions at all. It just clusters symptoms and theorizes mental illnesses with which to label us and sends us on our way.

One sign that something was very, very wrong was the absence of books on my nightstand. I could barely read but forced myself to when I had to grade papers or comment on students' work. My eyes couldn't focus on the words on the page: *sabotage, mine, are, hour.* The marks seemed random: commas strewed, apostrophes dangling, dashes dashed. It took a month, but I figured out that if I listened to the audio version of a book with the book in front of me, I could keep track. Following along helped still the words on the page, place them, order them beside and between the correct punctuation marks to gather meaning.

Periods were the easiest to find. Those pronounced dots at the bottom of a line at the end of a sentence signal a contained thought: *Going off the drug was going to kill me.* Or an idea: *I kept going because it would be better once I was off the drug.* Or a declaration: *It was their fault. It was his fault. It was my fault.* The period orders. It comprehends.

Aristophanes of Byzantium invented it. The ancient Romans ignored it. When the seventh-century scholar Archbishop Isidore of Seville resurrected it, it maintained its shape (.) and position at the top of the line. According to J. H. Chauvier's *Treatise on Punctuation*, it was monks who provided the period's next evolution. As scribes of the Christian church, monks had to write quickly. They figured out that the Romans' way of writing in all caps without spaces or marks wasn't perhaps the most efficient. First came the practice of cursive (Latin for *running*) in which letters were connected, so the monks didn't have to lift their writing instruments from the page. They used a dot between each word and the *periodus*, a break indicated by three dots, to show where one thought ended and another began. The dot between words was replaced by a simple space, and the *periodus*, which started to appear under the final word, eventually assumed its place at the bottom of the line and the end of a sentence.[54]

Archbishop Isidore and those monks returned clarity to us. Understanding. They gave us back a sense of boundaries, limits. A place to say, *No more.*

———

But there was more, like the night I was in the bath—the water so hot it turned my skin red—trying to sweat my withdrawal symptoms into the clear bathwater, hoping to watch them drain.

They didn't, not in the bath, not while I put on pajamas and brushed my teeth and washed my face with soap, forgetting to rinse it with water. Not while I was in bed, listening to the pouring rain, desperate for sleep. Not when lightning flashed; not when a thunderclap reverberated in my brain, shocking the resting withdrawal symptoms to life. Not when my brain felt as though it were undoing itself, coming apart.

11

On Suicidal Ideation

At our next appointment, Dr. M cocked his head to the side and looked at me. On his desk behind him was his usual can of LaCroix Naturally Essenced Sparkling Water. He asked how I was doing.

His voice sounded far away. It felt as if the big gray couch was starting to swallow me. "I can't take it."

He turned to the LaCroix can and edged his finger under the tab.

I begged him to let me go back on the SSRI.

He reminded me of the damage it would do long-term to stay on it: a possible manic episode, rapid cycling.

Something seemed wrong, not about what he was saying but with the black file cabinet in the corner. Both drawers were open halfway. Papers stuck out of the file folders as if trying to escape. "The shudders and shivers. My thoughts. The nightmares—they're too much."

"Your body and mind are reacting, not being damaged," he said.

I thought again of the morning I first took the SSRI, standing at the kitchen counter, the pill bottle open in front of me. How a shaft of sunlight came through the window. How much I believed the SSRI would make me better. Now, *better* was no longer in the equation; I needed the SSRI. "Please, let me go back on it."

He lifted the tab of the LaCroix can. The carbonation released with a hiss. "Give it time."

The "essence" of grapefruit reached me—strong and acidic.

––––––

Someone once told me that hope is deadly. It's expectation (the certainty that something will happen) mixed with desire (want). But nothing in life is certain and our expectations are so rarely met, which means that hope is actually a kind of tormenting want, something akin to what the Greek mythological figure Tantalus experienced when he was condemned to be forever thirsty and hungry in Hades, the fruit on the branches of a nearby tree always out of reach.

Still, we equate hope with strength. Its symbol is an anchor. Sometimes, it's a butterfly. Occasionally, a dove.

In positive psychology circles, hope exists on a spectrum. Real hope blends optimism into reality. False hope is the deluded belief in the impossible.

I had hope. Not firm-anchored hope. Not flitting-butterfly hope. Not free-as-a-dove hope. False hope that one medication or treatment for *my bipolar* would be the answer.

––––––

A month later, I sat on the swallowing gray couch in Dr. M's office. He clapped his hands almost enthusiastically. We were nearing the end of the SSRI titration. Soon, I'd be off it.

The withdrawal symptoms had seemed to build, climax, and now scraped along. Gone were the hallucinations, paranoia, sweating, agitation, nightmares, the brain shivers and shudders and zaps, but not the anxiety, confusion, irritability, insomnia, or crying spells, which seemed minor in comparison.

He strongly recommended I start on lithium. "The gold standard for bipolar."

I knew little about it aside from the Nirvana song of the same name (though Kurt Cobain said the song was about the power of religion, not the drug, to save a person from suicide[1]) and Kay Redfield Jamison's unbridled praise of it, which bordered on evangelizing.

I said I wanted to try other, more natural approaches first.

He raised his eyebrows. "Lithium's natural."

This was true. It rests below hydrogen and above sodium on the periodic table. "I just want to try a few more things first."

———

There wasn't much left to try. I'd heard of cognitive behavioral therapy, which was touted by some for its effectiveness in helping to treat many DSM diagnoses, including bipolar.[2] The treatment primarily involves filling out worksheets. In doing so, the patient becomes able to manage her thoughts and establish healthier behaviors.

CBT didn't come naturally. At the time, I believed that psychiatric medications were the best and most necessary treatment for my diagnosis. By then, I was on three: the SSRI (which I still wasn't off), a benzodiazepine (for the brain zaps and panic attacks caused by withdrawal), and the anticonvulsant/mood stabilizer lamotrigine. Lithium, the miracle mood stabilizer, would make four.

I read books on CBT and did the worksheets—lots and lots of worksheets. It was somewhat helpful. *Feeling Good*, by David Burns—a Stanford psychiatrist who was a student of Aaron Beck, the father of CBT—was the most convincing of CBT's powers. Burns's books popularized CBT in the 1980s. The CBT workbooks made me aware of my black-and-white thinking; the way I overgeneralized and catastrophized; and how I jumped to conclusions, mentally filtered the negative in most situations, and thought I knew what other people were thinking. But it didn't lessen my symptoms or change how I was functioning.

It did make me consider taking lithium. I'd thought CBT would be presented as the alternative to medication. But Burns wrote that bipolar disorder (*my* diagnosis) may require mood-stabilizing medications such as lithium.[3]

CBT also made me believe even more strongly in my bipolar diagnosis. Part of it was that CBT used the same labels—*major depression*, *anxiety disorder*, *post-traumatic stress disorder*—which made them seem even more real. Everyone seemed to agree they were valid.

But I was still wary of lithium. I agreed to try Tegretol, another anti-convulsant used as a mood stabilizer. It seemed fine at first. We started with a small dose. After three days, he upped it dramatically. It didn't seem right, but he was the expert. I stood at the counter in the morning and at night, three mornings and nights in a row, and swallowed the shockingly large beige pill.

It made me so ill I couldn't move. I emailed to tell Dr. M. Later, when he called, his voice was taut and angry. He said we'd discuss it at our next session.

Standing at his office door to greet me, he looked annoyed. I entered, feeling as though I'd done something terribly wrong. He sat at his desk. The LaCroix can stood by the phone. Still weak, I lowered myself onto the gray couch.

He said the pills weren't making me sick. Even if they were, I shouldn't have made my email sound like it was an emergency. I should give the medication a chance.

"To do what?" I asked.

He turned away and opened the LaCroix. "To work."

We spoke of finding my next medication as if it were urgent. Certainly, an episode was imminent. Depressive or manic (who knew for sure?), it was weeks, maybe days away. If I wanted to prevent it, I'd listen to him and take lithium.

I asked again about the side effects. He said my thyroid would probably stop working, but I didn't need it anyway. There'd be weight gain. Maybe acne. Toxicity was an issue[4] but "not a big one."

"We'll check your lithium levels," Dr. M said. I must have looked worried because he followed this with an impatient "It's fine," as if to say, *Stop making such a big deal out of it.*

It all made sense. Very sick people need very powerful drugs. I was very sick. I had to treat my bipolar. "Okay, I'll take it."

He raised his eyebrows. His mouth twitched, then curved into a smile. This, he said, was a breakthrough in my recovery.

———

Lithium's history[5] is storied.[6] In the early nineteenth century, it was thought of as a tonic prescribed to remedy gout and rheumatism, and by the end of the century literally flowed like water: companies advertised "Lithia Water" and boasted of its lithium content, billing it as a remedy for nearly everything. It was a key ingredient in 7Up (yes, the soft drink), promoted as a way to have energy, enthusiasm, and avoid a hangover. But when it was marketed as a salt substitute, it earned an FDA warning after it was said to have contributed to the deaths of multiple people.[7] Because of the risk of toxicity, the FDA didn't approve it as a bipolar medication until 1974. The World Health Organization included it on its list of essential medicines. In academic journals, it was alternately cast as a miracle drug, a placebo, or a poison.

———

I had my blood drawn and my levels monitored at a diagnostic lab across the street from Dr. M's office. Over the months, it became routine. I'd check in with the bored receptionist behind the counter, sit in the waiting area, and half-watch *Ellen* or some other daytime talk show on the TV mounted on the wall.

The threat of toxicity was real. I could end up in a coma with brain damage or dead. Possible side effects included tremors, increased urination, thirst, diarrhea, vomiting, weakness, blurred vision, ringing in the ears, thyroid dysfunction, and kidney failure.

During one appointment, after my name was called, I followed the lab technician to the back room and sat in the chair. She tourniqueted the plastic tubing around my bicep. I looked away as the needle pricked my skin, clocking the seconds until it was over and the nurse pressed the gauze to my skin and told me to keep pressure on it.

I later walked down Wabash under the L train. The light-headedness came on fast, followed by a wave of nausea and the certainty that I was going to throw up. I went to the curb, rested my hand on the hood of a car, leaned over, and dry heaved. And again.

The nausea and dry heaving didn't go away, not for two months. Two months, all day long, with barely a moment of relief, two months of being so nauseated I gagged and dry heaved and sometimes had trouble walking a block. Two months of eating mostly saltines and yogurt and ginger. Even teaching became strenuous.

Any woman who's been pregnant would have glanced at me sidelong: *Yeah, I'll tell you about nausea.* But in pregnancy, at least, nausea is a rite of passage in the gestation process that leads to a new life—the miracle of their own progeny. This led nowhere.

I asked Dr. M if the lithium might be causing it.

He said it wasn't. My nausea would pass.

———

It didn't. I made an appointment with a gastroenterologist. Waiting in the examination room, I filled out a brief form. At the bottom was a series of boxes to check with each symptom filed under a category: *Circulatory, Muscular, Allergy, Digestive,* and . . . *Psychiatric.*

After one firm knock on the door, the doctor entered. She was young, mid-thirties. Her blond hair was tousled in a ponytail. Her pug nose made her seem disagreeable, but her warmth was genuine, signaled by the skin around her eyes that creased when she smiled.

We went through my symptoms. She listened, asked questions, and took notes. After an examination, she speculated three causes for my complaints: anxiety, cyclical vomiting, or psychiatric-medication interactions.

I asked if lithium could be the cause.

"No," she said. "But it might be the anticonvulsant."

"The lamotrigine? I've been on it for years."

"A new medication can trigger different side effects in an old medication."

"So it is the lithium."

"In a sense," she said. "But we can't be sure that's what it is."

When I told Dr. M it might be the lithium after all, he said—matter-of-factly—that it wasn't. I asked if it might be. He insisted it wasn't.

"She said it might be."

"It will pass."

———

Of course I considered stopping the lithium without telling Dr. M. If I had, I'd have joined the many patients with serious mental illnesses who exhibit noncompliant behavior (NCB) by not taking their medications as prescribed. (Some researchers prefer the term *nonadherence* because noncompliance makes it sound as if the patient has no agency.[8]) It's common. One review found that NCB rates among people being treated for chronic conditions could be as high as 77 percent. NCB contributes to higher rates of relapse, hospitalizations, emergency room visits, substance abuse, work absences, and suicidal behavior. It also contributes to higher health care costs.[9]

NCB is a passive act of resistance, which isn't to say it isn't damaging. It's a betrayal of the physician-patient relationship. And it's dangerous. It can sometimes look like carelessness. Or irresponsibility. Or willfulness. Or hopelessness.

But I kept taking the lithium—swallowing the white pill—partly because I'm a rule follower (someone reading this has probably already diagnosed me with perfectionism) and partly because I'd finally stopped taking the SSRI and hoped (*hoped*) I was finally on the right medications. So I took the lithium. I took it even though it was making me ill.

———

That summer, while my mother was out of town, I went for my usual walk along the lake. It felt like I was in a dream. The world around me seemed gauzy, the way the pages of my books had in high school. Gauzier: the beachgoers' voices were muffled, their laughter seemed to crackle, the waves seemed to froth as they crested.

A thought came: *I could just end it.* Then: *pills, water.* Then the image of me in the water and all of it gone. I don't know how long I stood there before I thought of my mother. I couldn't do that to her. She'd blame herself.

I told Dr. M. It seemed like the right thing to do. He was my psychiatrist, the man keeping me from breaking down. I couldn't hide anything from him.

He upgraded my diagnosis to bipolar I and said that because I'd been suicidal and had a plan, it was necessary for me to be in a partial hospitalization program (PHP).

"What's that?" I asked.

Of the four levels of care—inpatient (the hospital), residential, PHP, and intensive outpatient (IOP)—PHP was like being in the hospital without having to spend the night.

I'd also have to stop seeing him—this was protocol—and rely on the therapists and psychiatrists in the PHP. He asked if I thought he was abandoning me. I said I did. He said he wasn't: I was ill and needed help.

As a clinician, Dr. M wasn't supposed to be able to predict if I'd attempt to end my life, only to recognize if my risk for suicide had increased. Often that comes down to whether a patient has a plan. But researchers have found that passive suicidal ideation (no plan) can, in some cases, be as clear an indicator of risk for suicide as active suicidal ideation. "Ideator status" (passive versus active) can change during a depressive episode.[10] Having a "desire for death" and a plan to end one's life indicate similar risk rates for suicide—having both is, of course, the riskiest of all.[11]

Dr. M's conclusions as to my risk for suicide likely would have been influenced by the 1979 suicidal ideation scale developed by Aaron Beck and Maria Kovacs. On the scale, he would have given my desire, seriousness, deception, and the availability of my chosen method a score between zero and two.[12] My "predisposition to suicide" would be factored in. I probably would have come out a two: marital status—unmarried women are at a higher risk than married ones (two), triggering events (a two—history of relationship instability, chronic worrier, perfectionist), symptomatic presentation (two—I was bipolar and agitated), presence of hopelessness (two), frequency of suicidal thinking (two—often, intense, and for long periods), previous suicidal behavior (one—never actually tried), impulsivity (one), and protective factors that might prevent me (zero—my reasons for living were few beyond writing and feeling an outsize need to be there for my students and teach my next class).

But he never disclosed how he assessed my condition. And I (foolishly) never asked.

———

On my first day in the PHP, I arrived five minutes early. The reception area was oppressively air conditioned. I wasn't teaching that summer and had the time and insurance to pay the thousand-dollar-a-day fee. As soon as I entered, I wanted to leave.

The director of the program welcomed me. She was young and nice without being saccharine. As we walked to her office, goose bumps prickled my skin. More goose bumps. More cold rooms. My mind twisted with thoughts of how sick I was. I had to be. I was there.

After the intake, the director showed me to the kitchen and the refrigerator available to patients. I was *a patient*. When she dropped me at my assigned group room, she asked if I needed anything. I wanted to say, *Yes, to leave.*

Instead, I sat in one of the chairs that had been formed into a circle. As other patients arrived, I eyed the door. The more people there, the easier it would be to slip out. A woman about my age with dark curly hair entered. Then a young man who might have been one of my students. Then a woman who looked to be in her twenties with a pixie cut. No one spoke. Most sat and pulled out binders.

A whiteboard covered either wall. A classroom. I could be a student. No problem.

The two facilitators arrived—a young guy and a youngish woman, both of whom walked with the confident air of the well-adjusted. The woman gave me a binder filled with handout after handout of CBT worksheets. In the back were some on dialectical behavioral therapy (DBT). Originally designed for people with borderline personality disorder (BPD), DBT teaches patients how to "live in the moment" and regulate their emotions.

The facilitators took turns lecturing us on how to treat thoughts as if they weren't necessarily "true." *I can't do this* and *I'm not good enough* and *It's their fault* were just propositions put forth by the mind. I took thorough notes.

During lunch, I organized my binder for easy reference. We were later assigned homework. That night, I went home and shared with my mother what I'd learned. She looked as hopeful as I felt.

The next day, I saw the in-house psychiatrist, Dr. V. He was beyond caring. His dark, enthusiastic eyes were those of a man who genuinely wanted to serve every patient as best he could.

I had my final meeting with Dr. M that afternoon. He said he'd spoken to Dr. V.

"And?" I asked. "What did he say?"

Dr. M smiled. "He said, 'Wow, she's really bipolar.'"

The PHP was remarkably undramatic. Twenty or so patients filled the room each morning. In the afternoons, we were divided up into smaller groups of four or five. Most of the patients were white, more women than men. They had the insurance or the monetary support to be there. Those I talked to were on paid leave from their jobs.

Two patients told me they "were" bipolar I. (They didn't say they had it; they said they were it.) None of them had symptoms like mine. None was on the same medications. Yet we all supposedly had the same diagnosis.

Art therapy was my least favorite part. For someone who prefers not to draw or be spoken to like a six-year-old, each day having to sit around a table and paint my emotions or cut pictures out of magazines to create a vision of my perfect home was a little hell.

My fellow patients seemed not to mind. Some had actually volunteered to be there "to work on themselves." I sympathized with them. Many were clearly in pain. But every morning on my commute to the program and on my way home I passed people living on the street, an estimated 25 percent of whom were most likely struggling with serious mental illness and as many as 45 percent with mental health conditions.[13] PHPs are another result of deinstitutionalization. For those with insurance and means, they're the community centers that never were, meant to shelter those who need more than a psychiatrist's and therapist's help and to transition those who've been hospitalized or in residential care. All of it made me question who was getting help and who wasn't.

————

The next time I saw Dr. V, he recommended an antipsychotic in addition to the lithium. An antipsychotic would help with my anxiety now that I was off the SSRI. It was often used to "complement" mood stabilizers like the ones I was on. It would bring my medications back up to four.

He said he'd consulted Dr. M, who'd agreed. The side effects were many: agitation, anxiety, constipation, dry mouth, insomnia. And massive weight gain (thirty to a hundred pounds), which could lead to diabetes and high cholesterol, which could lead to other major health issues, which could lead to death. And nausea, which I was already battling. And tardive dyskinesia—jerky, involuntary movements like waving one's arms or jutting one's tongue out over and over—a side effect that wouldn't necessarily go away even after I stopped the drug.

"And akathisia," Dr. V said.

"What's that?"

"Extraordinarily rare," he said, his chin jutting slightly as if to emphasize the point.

I asked what it was.

"Basically, restlessness."

Restlessness didn't seem that bad.

So I filled the prescription and returned to my mother's apartment. Standing at the kitchen counter, I swallowed the pill—a beacon of hope.

————

I didn't ask why I was prescribed an antipsychotic without ever having been psychotic. The derealization and depersonalization I'd experienced were considered dissociative, not psychotic, disorders. I didn't ask because Dr. V presented it as the professional standard.[14] Nothing to worry about. The FDA approved some antipsychotics to treat bipolar but not Rexulti, which I was given. It hadn't been approved to treat anxiety or insomnia either, but psychiatrists prescribed it for those, too.[15]

The FDA approves drugs for specific illnesses but allows physicians to prescribe them "off-label" for just about anything. Its reasoning is difficult to fathom, almost Alice-in-Wonderland-ish in its logic. The FDA website tells patients it's up to the physician's discretion: "From the FDA perspective, once the FDA approves a drug, health care providers generally may prescribe the drug for an unapproved use when they judge that it is medically appropriate for their patient."[16] Why, then, go through the hassle of approving a drug for a specific use in the first place?

Without off-label prescribing, antipsychotics would have been limited to the small number of people who actually experienced psychosis. Antipsychotics are prescribed for depression, anxiety, ADHD, childhood conduct disorders, even insomnia.[17]

On the gray market, pharmaceutical companies, like Pfizer and others, make billions from off-label prescriptions.[18] Though it is prohibited by the FDA, some make claims in direct-to-consumer, ask-your-doctor campaigns that fail to tell viewers that the drugs they may take will be for an unapproved indication and unapproved age group in an unapproved dose and unapproved form of administration. The *Mayo Clinic Proceedings* journal encourages off-label drug use.[19] Patient-advocacy groups—like the National Alliance on Mental Illness, which received $23 million from pharmaceutical companies between 2006 and 2008;[20] the Depression and Bipolar Support Alliance, which the *Los Angeles Times* reported got half its funding from pharma;[21] and Children and Adults with Attention-Deficit/Hyperactivity Disorder, which reportedly received nearly a quarter of its funding from pharma—tell the public that taking off-label medications is safe and "helpful."[22]

Helpful means "of service or assistance." Without data, studies, or any basis for making such claims, what service and assistance could off-label prescribing provide?

―――――

Three nights later, I sat on my bed in my room rocking back and forth. It had been that way for an hour or more. I sat but not with any sense of leisure; I wanted out of my skin. Occasionally, I stood and paced. When I stopped pacing, I continued to move, shifting my weight from one foot to the other or lifting one leg and the next over and over again, marching in place. When I sat, I crossed and uncrossed my legs.

It was like someone else was inside me, moving me. I rocked. I stood again. I paced. I marched. I rocked.

Then a violent agitation seized me. Dark and aggressive.

I called Dr. M, barely hearing the options for which number to press to leave a message. My hands shook. I spoke fast. To the wrong person, I might have sounded manic. After I left the message, I ran to the bathroom for a bout of diarrhea. I returned to my room and marched in place.

When Dr. M returned my call, I explained again, talking very fast. As I did, I sat on the edge of the bed, tapping my foot, crossing and uncrossing my legs.

"You may be having a reaction," he said, sounding concerned. "Akathisia."

Turns out akathisia isn't "extraordinarily rare"; it is, in fact, a common side effect of antipsychotic drugs.[23] Estimates range from 10 to 45 percent of those who take such medications are affected.[24] It's considered one of the most dangerous side effects because it can cause such anguish as to drive a person to suicide, which I took the pill to prevent.

Dr. M and Dr. V lowered the dose and put me on a regimen of Benadryl. Eventually, the akathisia lessened. They recommended I try a different antipsychotic, Vraylar. I said yes out of the hope that it would "work"—though I no longer knew what that meant. The akathisia returned, just as brutal. They said they could only lower the dose, reminding me how sick I was and that I needed to stay on an antipsychotic. It seemed impossible and senseless. I didn't agree, but I didn't argue either.

Hopeless is defined as "having or feeling no hope," as if *no hope* were an emotion. To be hopeless is to despair. It's a state of desperation beyond want and need. A kind of void with no way out. In positive psychology, *no hope* means helplessness; *lost hope*, resignation.

Though suicide can be an act of desperation, it also signals a loss of hope. Someone who's suicidal is left without the expectation of a future, without desire, and without the two in combination. To a person experiencing suicidal ideation, John Locke's statement about hope would feel like it was written in a foreign language: "Hope is that pleasure in the mind, which everyone finds in himself, upon the thought of a probable future enjoyment of a thing which is apt to delight him." *Everyone? Probable future? Delight?* Alexander Pope's famous statement would be even more unintelligible: "Hope springs eternal in the human breast." *Eternal?*

My suicidality—being actively suicidal—was filled with the desire to live. Because if I only wanted to die, I wouldn't have been suicidal; I would have been dead.

———

I was discharged from the PHP because I had to teach. The director didn't want me to go. I asked if everyone there was independently wealthy. She asked if I could file for short-term disability leave. No, neither of the universities where I taught offered disability leave to part-time professors, as if only full-time employees fell ill.

My first night teaching after being in the PHP, my students sat at the tables shaped into a square, seminar-style. I stood at the whiteboard with my back to them. The marker felt strange in my hand. My legs shook. It was like coming to work when you think you've recovered from the flu—a long flu—only to find you're still sick and regular life demands too much.

I put the name of the course on the whiteboard: *ENG 208: Writing and Reading Creative Nonfiction.* The letters were in the correct order, made into words that made meaning we could all understand.

Canceling the class and claiming illness wasn't an option. I could, of course, but with the shakiness and strangeness came a need to be with students, to be of use.

I turned to them. Like so many of my creative writing classes, it was mostly made up of women. I smiled and as I did, the smile became genuine.

One student, Katie, was so eager to learn I felt like I was learning from her. There's always at least one in a class, a student hungry not just for information or knowledge but understanding, integrating the class into her very being. Her engagement wasn't grade driven; she wasn't skimming the surface. Her hunger came from somewhere deep, a place few students find mainly because no one else has it to give, so it has to come from them.

Soon, Katie and the others were all I thought about. The chair I sat on felt real. The pen in my hand, too. The sentences on the handouts I passed out made sense. The three hours sped by.

But as they packed their things to leave, fear sank inside me. Katie stayed after class to talk more about the essay we'd read—an excerpt from Claudia Rankine's *Citizen*. We'd run out of time just as we started to discuss the section called "Stop and Frisk," in which Rankine writes about racial profiling. Katie said something about the characters being forced into silence. I wanted to hear her, but her voice sounded so far away.

————

I've never understood mental-illness memoirists and bloggers who say they had a "love affair" with suicide. Suicidality is a vortex. It's deafening and silent. Empty and full of horror. The darkest place I've ever touched.

On the first autumn morning of the year, the weather app on my phone said fifty-eight degrees. Outside my window, the wind blew—no, ripped through the trees. A motorcycle roared past my window. I imagined the man driving it dressed in yellow leather. My gym bag—with the pills in it—sat on my bed.

People describe suicidality as linear. There's a reason, a plan. But it's not that orderly. Although the akathisia was gone, my thoughts had been spinning for three days. Sometimes, they shouted. Sometimes, they were viciously "helpful," offering new suicidal thoughts—other methods, different timings, new locations.

I left my mother's apartment and pushed through the front door of the building and onto the street. Blue sky. Sun. Pedestrians. Down the block came the little white dog I disliked and its owner whom I'd never spoken to. The crackling grind of an iron balcony being soldered on the apartment building across the street made me hunch over.

I saw Dr. M that afternoon. With the pills still in my bag, I sank onto the gray couch and started to cry. I wanted so much not to want to die. I mentioned the pills. Once it was out, I couldn't take it back.

Second time. Clear plan. He asked if I wanted him to call an ambulance or if I could get to the hospital myself.

———

The security guard at the emergency room took my belongings, cataloged them, and locked them up—pills inside. She was genuine, almost apologetic as she directed me to sit in a chair with the other "SIs"—those with suicidal ideation. Security guards watched us to make sure we didn't try to harm ourselves or leave.

The SI next to me rubbed the stubble on his chin. His eyes were knowing, like he'd been there before. His flannel shirt was clean, his khaki pants dirty, his Timberlands untied. A nurse in dark blue scrubs came up and asked him questions: *Are you suicidal? Have you taken anything? Have you cut yourself? Do you hear voices? Are you seeing things that aren't there?* He answered: Yes, no, no, hesitant yes, no.

The nurse asked, *Are you homeless?* "Yes," he answered.

She asked, *Do you have allergies?* "Yes," he said with authority, "Haldol."

It's pretty much impossible to be allergic to Haldol, an antipsychotic that's the stuff of nightmares.[25] It's potent and can produce a zombie-like effect.[26] That SI knew the drill and how to handle himself.

The nurse told me to go into the bathroom to put on a gown. Then she led me to a triage area with a curtain that couldn't be drawn so the security guards could still watch me.

Two new male SIs arrived, one in Velcro restraints because he'd been brought in by police, the other passed out on his gurney.

After an hour and fifteen minutes (I stared at the clock), a nurse came in. She looked so young she could have been thirteen. She took my vitals. Then she struggled to get the vials of blood they needed. The doctor, she said, would be in soon to finish my medical check. Then, finally, a psychiatrist would see me about being admitted.

The sound of a woman screaming incoherently came from down the hall. Her words were a jumble of gasps and curses and "get your hands off me" and "someone's gotta help." The doctors in the station across from me discussed her loudly. They debated the options for treatment. The woman's screams turned to howls. One doctor said something about an injection. Another confirmed: Haldol and Ativan. The woman screamed. The doctors moved out of view. Within ten minutes, all was quiet again.

Four hours later, I was still waiting to see a psychiatrist. The two men and the sedated woman were ahead of me in line. Later, I'd learn fourteen people were waiting to see the psychiatrist that day.

An hour later, the psychiatrist still hadn't shown. Finally, I asked what was going to happen and found out there were no beds at that hospital, no beds at any of the closest four hospitals with psych wards in the Chicago area. I begged to be discharged and—with the permission of Dr. M and my mother agreeing to assume responsibility—was released on the condition I enter a PHP the following week. I was asking them to make an exception because the hospital was liable for me.

That was the counterpart to the PHPs that resulted from deinstitutionalization. Two of the men, assuming they were admitted, might be transferred to the state hospital. The woman? Who knew. The man in restraints would likely be rerouted to the Cook County Jail.

That night, I sat at my desk. I'd been released to a warm apartment and a loving mother and had access to care. What about the men and the woman in the emergency room? What had happened to them?

———

Few understand the power of the semicolon. It's our most intimidating punctuation mark, one people either avoid or cling to, whether they know how to use it properly or not. It's an unnecessary punctuation mark, except in the case of a list with commas. To me, it demands a mastery of finality (the period) and continuity (the comma).

That wasn't its original function. It's said to have first appeared in Venice in 1494 as a fusion of the comma and the colon.[27] The printer and publisher Aldus Manutius—who also brought us the comma—created and commissioned it to offer readers and writers a way to pause longer than the comma but not end. It was born out of the Italian literati's zeal for experimentation and invention.

Its rules weren't uniform. Like so many punctuation marks that European printers used during the fifteenth, sixteenth, and seventeenth centuries, its usage was left up to the individual.

By the nineteenth century, it was no longer a typographical mark that indicated a pause or could be placed in a sentence for effect. Its rules became more rigid: It joined related clauses. Historian and philosopher Cecelia Watson writes that this arose out of a shift in the way grammar was thought of at the time. Grammar and punctuation were no longer left up to the individual; they had "general principles."[28] They could be categorized and classified. (Perhaps ironically, in terms of mental illness diagnoses, this was the Kraepelin era, a time marked by the ordering and classification of mental disorders.)

That day in my room, I hadn't yet heard of Project Semicolon, an anti-suicide campaign that, in 2013, transformed the semicolon from a challenging-to-use punctuation mark into a symbol of strength.[29] The organization that led the campaign traced the semicolon back to its original function: as a way to pause. The semicolon could help those in a moment of hopelessness pause instead of ending their lives. The organization's slogan read, *Your story isn't over*. People tattooed semicolons on their wrists, backs, and chests in solidarity and posted photos of themselves on social media, where Project Semicolon gained a massive following. At the time, the organization's home page told me, "[A] semicolon represents a sentence the author could have ended, but chose not to. The sentence is your life and the author is you."

III

12

⚫︎

"Sick"

It came as a shock: *DSM diagnoses are invalid? Unreliable? Invented? Not based in science? Not medically sound?* How could the six diagnoses I'd received—and all DSM diagnoses—be just words in a book?

That would mean I should have put them in quotation marks—scare quotes. Scare quotes signify doubt: "anorexia," "OCD," "ADHD," "anxiety disorder," "major depression," "bipolar disorder." Scare quotes (sometimes called sneer or shudder quotes) tell the reader that the term inside the quotation marks should be taken with a healthy dose of skepticism.

No one knows exactly how and when the practice of putting quotes around words to warn the reader against taking the word at face value started. According to the *Oxford English Dictionary*, the term *scare quotes* first appeared in print in 1956. The OED describes them as "disassociating the user from the expression." The linguist David Crystal writes that scare quotes "tell the reader that they can't take [the words inside the quotation marks] for granted, but must look for special meaning in the mind of the writer."[1] Scare quotes could have saved me from believing in the diagnoses found in "psychiatry's bible" as if they were the gospel truth.

At the very least, those diagnoses should be in regular quotation marks; they're the written record of ideas discussed by the DSM's authors. Quotation marks show that someone is speaking. Most grammarians agree they evolved from the diple, a typographical mark that looks like an arrowhead (>).[2] They then transformed into double commas at the bottom of the line („). By the nineteenth century, they appeared as the elevated, inverted double commas we know today (") and were used to distinguish what one person (usually a fictional character) says from another.

With them, things might have turned out differently.

————

On my last day at my next PHP, which I ended up in after the previous suicidal episode, I walked down the hallway past the many therapists' offices. This PHP was different—more traditional with lots and lots of therapy. The hallway was filled with the familiar whirr of the white-noise machines on the floor outside each office to prevent passersby from hearing what was being said in a session.

The first activity that morning was "Skill." It was a lot like it sounds. A therapist or two would teach us a skill that would, ostensibly, help us function better. Many of the skills came from Acceptance and Commitment Therapy (ACT), yet another CBT-based treatment that told me to accept my emotions, observe my experiences objectively, be present, clarify my values, and set goals.

In the room where Skill was held, I joined the others on one of the soft couches arranged in a circle. No one spoke. The windows looked onto the opposite building into offices, giving us a view into the world outside the PHP, a world of people typing and conferencing and collegially laughing.

The two therapists facilitating that morning's session came in. Both were nice, but over the months I'd been there, they, like all the therapists, had remained standoffish, not even learning our names. They handed out a worksheet with a bull's-eye circle on it. My inner A-student kicked in. As directed, I filled in each ring, deciding where in my life I was hitting the bull's-eye and where I was on the outer rim.

After Skill, I met with my therapist for my exit interview. Her office was tiny and softly lit. The one window looked onto a brick wall. She smiled when I entered. I sat in the faux fur chair opposite her desk. She was blond and sunny and laughed a lot.

I didn't just complain to her; she was the first therapist I had who acted primarily as a resource. She'd met with my mother, my sister, and me to help us map out an emergency plan for when (*when*, not *if*) I was in crisis. That PHP didn't have a psychiatrist on-site, so I saw Dr. M for my medications but only a couple of times during the four months I was there. She'd asked about my relationship with him and if I was getting the treatment I needed. I said, "Yes." She looked at me sidelong, obviously hearing the hesitation in my voice.

We talked about my time in the program. It had been a luxury. Although I was still teaching while in it, my primary focus was the program. I learned and applied the skills. In group therapy sessions, I vaguely processed what I viewed as my troubling thoughts and emotions.

And I took my *meds*. Not *med*, *meds*—plural, never singular. A cocktail of drugs. (*Polypharmacy* is the official term.) As part of the lingua franca of the PHP, *meds* were for those embedded in the mental health industrial complex, those on mood stabilizers and antipsychotics, those who cycled through hospitals and residential programs (referred to slangly as "reses") and PHPs and IOPs. *Meds* implied chronic. *Meds* implied severe side effects: obesity, kidney failure, tremors, tardive dyskinesia, diabetes. *Meds* implied the drug had as good a chance of damaging the body as it did of healing the brain.

On that final day in the PHP, I asked my therapist about my diagnosis. We worked together under the assumption that I had what my chart said I had: bipolar. I don't know what made me question it that day (truly, I don't), but I wanted her opinion. "Do you think I'm bipolar?"

She didn't respond for some time, looking at the ceiling, considering. "Well, I'm not the one who decides your diagnosis, but you've never seemed to have the classic bipolar symptoms, I guess."

I didn't ask what that meant; instead, I told her about the lingering effects of the SSRI withdrawal. They hadn't gone away. There was still anxiety, confusion, irritability, insomnia, and crying jags. "I don't know how else to stop them."

"What do you want to do?" she asked.

"Go back on the Zoloft."

She nodded. "Do you feel like you can talk to Dr. M about that yourself?"

"Sure," I said. "Of course."

When I reached the group therapy room, two other patients were there. They stared down at their phones. I took my usual spot on a couch in the corner. None of us spoke.

I felt in my pocket for the "Feelings Wheel" handout we'd been given. Folded, creased, and wearing at the edges, the handout showed a drawing of a circle sliced into slim pie pieces, each with its own emotion: *bored, sickened, worried, helpless, hesitant, affectionate, connected, curious, caring*. At the start of each group session, we had to go around and say our names and how we were feeling. I was either fine or not fine, okay or not okay, good or not-so-good. But *okay* and *not-so-good* weren't specific enough for the facilitators. So I studied the wheel and its emotions—*puzzled, frightened, safe, satisfied*—and considered which pulsed inside me: *anger, frustration*.

The others arrived, and the facilitator came in with his clipboard. We went through the usual: introducing ourselves, identifying our diagnoses, and saying how we felt.

"John. Schizoaffective. A little confused."

"Emma. Bulimia, anxiety disorder, bipolar II, PTSD. Sad."

For the first time, it struck me: We labeled ourselves with our diagnoses. We spoke them aloud as if swearing allegiance. "Sarah," I said. "Frustrated."

If I'd known how unsubstantiated the DSM diagnoses are, I might never have been in that room. Even bits and pieces, such as how the DSM-III was sold to the public as scientifically proven. Or how it was marketed not only to psychiatrists and researchers but also psychologists, social workers, insurance companies, government agencies, pharma, managed care facilities, medical students, school systems, disability agencies, courts, and the general public, who (for the most part) had no medical training.[3] Or how it was a boon to the financially floundering American Psychiatric Association. (The DSM-II brought in $1.27 million, the DSM-III $9.33 million, the DSM-III-R $16.65 million, and the DSM-IV $20 million.[4] The DSM-5 made the APA $20 million in its first year alone.)

I had no idea the later editions were created by task forces of psychiatrists, psychologists, and other health care professionals and that although that might sound like a lot of learned opinions and expertise, it isn't. Just twenty-eight people were on the DSM-5 task force. (To be fair, each member headed a work group of eight to fifteen others drawn from, according to the APA, a "diverse group of professionals," and consulted with "outside advisors."[5]) Or that the task force and work groups argued about each diagnosis based on theories when they didn't have data, which was most of the time.[6] Or that DSM diagnoses like social anxiety disorder pathologized the shy and oppositional defiant disorder stigmatized children of color like Darnell. Or that the DSM authors seemed hellbent on pathologizing normal activities by giving them labels like internet addiction disorder.[7]

If only I'd been aware of the "Feighner criteria" and its role in the making of the DSM-III. The Feighner criteria was a paper published by a group of research-oriented psychiatrists at Washington University in 1972.[8] It reenvisioned sixteen mental illnesses in terms of checklists of symptoms. (These are often referred to as "criteria sets" and the practice of relying on them "descriptive diagnosis.") Essentially, the paper tried to create a medical model of mental illness.[9]

Spitzer based the DSM-III on the Feighner criteria, which would have been fine except for at least three major stumbling blocks. First, the Feighner criteria defined only sixteen diagnoses; the DSM-III had ballooned to more than two hundred.[10] Second, the Feighner criteria was based on little empirical data, which means none of its diagnoses were valid either.[11] Third, it was meant for research purposes only—not for a psychiatrist diagnosing a patient in her office.[12]

Still, Spitzer was determined. A Feighner-criteria-inspired DSM-III would show that diagnoses based on symptom lists were medically sound and scientifically valid. It didn't. Essentially, the DSM-III reclustered symptoms, lowered thresholds, and presented divvied up and invented diagnoses as if doing so somehow made the manual scientific.

(Spitzer insisted that the DSM-III's diagnoses were, despite evidence to the contrary, sound. One argument he made was that they were more reliable than the DSM-II's, which wasn't saying much given that the DSM-II's were "appallingly poor."[13] He also cited the field trials that were conducted even though they weren't used to draft the DSM-III.[14])

The DSM-III served as the foundation for all DSMs to follow. The DSMs III-R and IV maintained the pretense that the manual was a work of science.[15] Work groups were formed. The literature was reviewed. Data sets were analyzed. Field trials were conducted. And 155 new diagnoses were added.

The DSM-5 professed to be even more "scientific" than the previous editions. It rebranded with the Arabic 5 instead of the Roman numeral *V* to signal a "new" approach that distinguished it from previous editions and said to the public, yes, this time, these diagnoses are scientific (for sure), even though they weren't.[16] Task forces and expensive field trials were set up to establish validity and reliability of the new disorders it planned to introduce. Allen Frances blasted them for asking "the wrong question, in the wrong way, in the wrong settings, and with an unrealistic timeline" and said the results were impossible to interpret.[17] This seemed not to matter. Diagnoses were changed and another 158 new diagnoses were added. Everyday behaviors like childhood temper tantrums (disruptive mood regulation disorder), mood changes before menstruation (premenstrual dysphoric disorder), and overeating (binge eating disorder, which states that anyone who has "binged" and felt bad about it once a week for the past three months is pathological) became mental illnesses.

As Paula Caplan, a psychologist and member of two DSM-IV work groups says, the DSM has little more than "a veneer" of science.[18] She writes: "The *DSM* authors diverge from responsible scientific practice . . . by designing and conducting studies in sloppy ways, by distorting their findings to make them look better than they are, and by not revealing some of their findings or revealing them too late."[19]

Maybe, if I knew that the DSM authors and supporters try and fail to justify the DSM by saying that although its diagnoses aren't valid, they're reliable (even though they're not) and that's all that matters, I wouldn't have been so quick to believe the diagnoses I'd been given. After all, agreement doesn't make something true. Caplan makes the analogy that we could all stand in a field and agree that a horse is a unicorn but that doesn't mean we've all seen a unicorn. (Another example: Just because Medieval doctors agreed on who they deemed witches, that didn't make those women witches.) Peter Tryer, professor of psychiatry and editor of the *British Journal of Psychiatry*, offers the example of ADHD. In studies, given the DSM-5's vague and extensive symptom list for ADHD, it would be easy enough to train those conducting the study (known as raters) to find high degrees of reliability. Tryer writes: "It is very important to realise [*sic*] that reliability in itself does not mean a disorder is better described or more valid in actually measuring what it purports to measure."[20] If only I'd been told how symptoms overlap. Someone with depression can feel anxious, someone with anxiety can experience severe depression, which would be fine (both people with the flu and meningitis can have a fever) if those with the same symptoms were diagnosed with the same disorder and those with the same diagnosis shared the same symptoms, which they don't. No "zone of rarity"—a clear marker between normal and abnormal—exists.

I might not have been in that room if I'd heard about the homosexuality controversy. Homosexuality was included in the DSM until the DSM-III in 1980. Its removal was a well-deserved triumph for gay rights activists that resulted from political and social pressure placed on the APA. In some ways, this brought DSM diagnoses into question: If the APA would (for the most part) erase a diagnosis from its pages for any reason other than scientific discovery, how many other diagnoses were equally unfounded? If I'd been educated about the DSM and its role in how we think and talk about mental illness, about its lowered thresholds and added diagnoses and manipulated punctuation and words that allow as many people as possible to be diagnosed regardless of whether they really have the disorder, about how its diagnoses aren't as reliable as psychiatrists want us to think[21] and not at all scientifically sound[22] and certainly not chronic, I wouldn't have wanted to end my life.

———

The primary color of Dr. M's new office was still gray. It had windows—large windows. The view was of Trump Tower. Gone was the old, swallowing couch; in its place was a stiff gray one. He'd increased the distance between his chair and the patient couch by about ten feet.

He wanted to talk about my time in the PHP, so we did. Soon, we were talking about my future and the prospect of me going on disability. Given my dire prognosis, things could possibly come to the point when I could no longer teach, maybe not even write.

Light reflected off the glassy surface of Trump Tower, causing the sun to glint in my eye. "I don't want to talk about this anymore."

His face twitched. "Okay, what would you like to talk about?"

I wanted to talk about my upcoming move. The apartment I'd found was in the rear of the building, away from the street. Without taking into account how small it was and the absence of any view, I'd signed the lease and arranged for a moving company.

Dr. M was surprised. "That was fast."

"It's necessary." This was true. My mother was starting to be weighed down from the strain of caring for me. She didn't say as much; she didn't have to. It was obvious in her wan, drawn face. I also felt the need to be in my own apartment.

He touched his well-coiffed hair and raised his eyebrows knowingly.

I waited until the end of our session to say that I wanted to go back on the SSRI.

He said he didn't think that was the best idea. I could "if I really wanted to," but I should at least try to give the other medications "a chance."

The discussion ended there. My chest tightened as I walked out of his office and down the carpeted hall, muttering, "He just loves the sound of his own voice."

———

Our sessions became passive-aggressive battles. Most were spent in tortuous discussions about the dynamics in our "relationship." I said I needed a doctor, not a relationship. He touched his gelled hair and raised his eyebrows.

Dr. M was a Freudian. Freud of the Oedipus complex and penis envy. Freud, who attributed so much to sex and for whom psychoanalysis wasn't a way to cure or help but *to probe* (pun intended). Freud, who believed that even analysis was an erotic relationship and had his daughter Anna discuss her masturbation fantasies with him. Freud, who was convinced that dysmenorrhea in women was caused by masturbation and that sexual organs were connected to the nose. His thirty-year-old patient Emma Eckstein almost died from a hemorrhage after he authorized a nasal operation to relieve her dysmenorrhea. Freud, who called the sexual life of women a "dark continent" and thought only men were moral because they weren't "castrated." Freud, whose many claims seem to have been picked from the sky. As Todd Dufresne wrote, "Arguably no other notable figure in history was so fantastically wrong about nearly every important thing he had to say."[23] Freud, who was also intolerant of dissent from those who didn't accept his theories, like Carl Jung and Alfred Adler.[24] Freud, who saw himself as a scientist though he extrapolated data based on a very small sample of patients or an *n of 1* (himself). Freud, who lied about the effectiveness of his talk-therapy cases and treated his own depression not with the talking cure but with cocaine.

Dr. M didn't approve of Freud in every respect. Neo-Freudians— including Freud's daughter Anna—have tried to redeem Freud's less ridiculous theories (though that's slim pickings) by acknowledging his shortcomings (which is a nice way of referring to them). Dr. M was Freudian in the sense that he believed the analyst had a special ability to discern in the patient what she couldn't know about herself without his assistance. My motives and feelings were hidden to me, requiring me to seek his help. Our sessions weren't a dialogue; they were built on a power structure and he had all the power. I talked, he listened, and in listening, he learned what I'd subjugated to my subconscious. He knew best.

———

The ironically named SELF-I scale measures how much you identify with having a mental illness. It was meant to assist those who may need help but don't pursue it because of stigma, socioeconomic factors, or prior treatment experiences.[25] In studies, it performs well, but it doesn't test for mental illness; it gauges if a person suspects mental illness could be a possibility.[26]

The SELF-I consists of five statements to which you indicate your level of agreement: *Don't agree at all, Don't agree, Undecided, Agree, Agree completely.* The first statement is too vague to be helpful: *Current issues I am facing could be the first signs of a mental illness.* What type of "issue" and how are issues signs of mental illness? The second is unclear: *The thought of myself having a mental illness seems doubtful to me.* Is the thought or the mental illness doubtful? The third is puzzling: *I could be the type of person that is likely to have a mental illness.* What "type of person" is that? The fourth is practical: *I see myself as a person that is mentally healthy and emotionally stable.* The final is really two statements separated by one of the most common punctuation errors—a comma splice: *I am mentally stable, I do not have a mental health problem.*

The comma should be a period. The two thoughts are separate. The two together beg so many questions. What's a "mental health problem"? Is it a DSM diagnosis? A Freudian neurosis? Emotional discomfort? What makes a person mentally stable or unstable? Does having a "mental health problem" mean a person isn't mentally stable? Does a mentally unstable person necessarily have a "mental health problem"?

At one time, I would have answered *Agree completely* to the first and third statements and *Don't agree at all* to the last two. I wouldn't have hesitated.

Trump Tower was clouded by an early-winter snow. I sat on the stiff couch. Dr. M sat across from me. The bottle of LaCroix sat on his desk: *Essenced. Flavored. Fake.*

I told him I wanted to see someone else for therapy. It seemed like the perfect solution: See him for my meds and find someone I could talk to.

He touched his well-gelled blond hair in a way that said that if I wasn't going to stay in my place, at least it would. He said I had to see him for both therapy and psychiatry.

"Is that your policy?" I asked.

"No," he said. "Someone with your diagnosis needs special care."

"Bipolar I?"

"Bipolar I with mixed features."

I didn't ask what that meant; instead, I said we should take a break.

He said this wasn't the right time, seeing as I'd just been discharged from a partial hospitalization program.

I stared out the window. Snowflakes swirled in the air. I said I needed to see someone new.

He shrugged, and with the movement of his shoulder, it was as though I'd fallen off a cliff. I pictured my pillbox at home and the nearly empty prescription bottles. Standing, I put on my coat. "I'm low on my medications. I'll need refills."

He said I should see my primary care physician.

She'd retired a month earlier. "I don't have one right now."

He said this was my decision.

Psychiatrist-less, physician-less, out of refills, and running low on medication, I left his office. It's hard to explain how impossible it seemed for me to find a new primary care physician let alone a new psychiatrist. The withdrawal would start again, this time from all my meds, all at once. It would be ferocious, making nausea and brain zaps and shivering seem enjoyable.

As I stepped onto the elevator, I realized what I'd done. What if Dr. M refused to see me again? What if he cut me off? I thought of going back and apologizing.

Once home, I sat at my desk in the blue tint of my computer screen and scrolled through page after internet page of doctor profiles. Rating sites like Zocdoc proved unhelpful in the extreme. What did "top" in the "Top Psychiatrists Near Me" list mean? What assessment was used to give a psychiatrist a 4.54-star rating? What did one star represent to the patients rating them? I made a list of three potential psychiatrists and called, making appointments with all of them.

———

The first psychiatrist's office broke with tradition. It was the size of three offices. The yellow walls should have been cheerier than they were. A desk stood in the corner. Most of the space was taken up by a large conference table and six chairs. We sat across from each other width-wise, which made it feel like a business meeting.

He was tall and wore a suit. His face was fleshy, and the skin on his cheeks hung down, reminding me of a basset hound. I barely remember the questions he asked because he seemed so depressed. If I hadn't been so worried and desperate, I'd have tried to cheer him up. At the end of our session, he agreed I was bipolar and said he wanted to increase the antipsychotic.

The second psychiatrist was thin with dark hair. I remember little about our appointment, except that he was my height. He must have agreed with the bipolar diagnosis, and I must not have liked him because I never considered seeing him again.

My last hope was a woman in her sixties whose chubby face made her seem youthful. In a shift that seemed to reverse our roles, she sat on the couch and I in the chair across from her. It made me feel at ease and in control.

As she asked me questions and seemed to listen attentively when

I answered, the soft white light of a floor lamp shone down on me. She was the one. She might even be able to refill my prescriptions that night. At the end of the session, she said she agreed with the bipolar diagnosis.

Fine, I thought. *Fine*.

I explained that I was almost out of my medications. She suggested I switch to an antipsychotic. The particular antipsychotic she mentioned had some of the worst side effects of any other on the market: weight gain of sometimes a hundred pounds, vomiting that never goes away, a platelet count that makes it hard for your blood to clot, tremors. It wasn't that she and I couldn't have discussed it, but it didn't bode well if that was her go-to med.

I had less than a handful of pills left.

———

My sister got a referral from a friend. Dr. R "squeezed me in" for an appointment. His office was on the twenty-second floor of an office building on the Magnificent Mile. The waiting room was nearly full of clients: a young man scrolling on his phone, a middle-aged woman talking on hers, an older man with glasses reading *Vanity Fair*.

When my name was called, I looked up to see a middle-aged man wearing a white button-down shirt and suit pants that had a sheen. He shook my hand and introduced himself. In his late forties, maybe early fifties, he was one of those men who oozed success and intelligence. I followed him down the hallway. His loafers looked too expensive to sully by walking in them.

His office had floor-to-ceiling windows that looked onto Michigan Avenue. The affluent view said that he was either very good at his job or at making money. The pedestrians on the street below looked like toy figures.

"Coffee?" he asked, pointing a finger in my direction. "Water?"

I said I was fine though I was thirsty. I just needed my prescriptions filled.

He directed me to sit in one of two plush leather armchairs that faced each other. Without a notepad or pen, he asked me questions. In response to my answers, he nodded—bouncy and affirming—as if to say, *I'm with you. Heard it before. Got it.* He seemed to have already decided everything about me.

When I told him about the suicidal episodes, he nodded, his chin jutting out: *Yup, heard it before. Got it.* I told him about the SSRI withdrawal and the akathisia; he asked about the timing of my suicidal episodes.

I asked if they were related.

He nodded ambiguously. "Could be."

The thirty minutes went fast. He stood and walked toward his glass top desk. "How are you on your meds?"

I told him I needed refills.

He opened his laptop and renewed my prescriptions. "We'll clean up the mess of meds you're on soon enough. When can you come in again?"

It was presumptuous of him to assume I wanted to see him again. I asked about my diagnosis.

He leaned back, nodded his bouncy nod, shrugged, and said, "I don't know."

"What?"

He smiled a strange, satisfied smile. "I don't know."

We scheduled my next appointment.

I walked down the hallway and rode the elevator to the lobby and walked out into the cold onto Chicago Avenue. My mind seemed to open: *I don't know.*

If he didn't know, none of them had known. They'd just *said.* I turned into the cold wind whipping off the lake and felt strong against it.

———

Not long after, I sat in my office opposite one of my students. Her blond hair was plaited. She was falling behind in my literature course, which was required for her major. The quarter was ending. She'd only attended four of ten classes. Her phone sat on my desk near her. Every thirty seconds or so the screen lit up with a notification.

She told me she was having trouble with all her classes. Her eyes teared up. She'd been given a new diagnosis: ADHD. "In high school, they said depression and put me on medication. It was awful."

I listened. She talked. As she did, her tears lessened.

We agreed for her to see her advisor and the dean of students and to take it from there. I recommended she consult the center for students with disabilities.

"Yeah, I guess I have a disability."

It wasn't my place to say otherwise.

———

At our next appointment, Dr. R still didn't level a diagnosis. We changed my meds. We'd titrate off the antipsychotic, up the benzo, and keep the rest the same.

The withdrawal symptoms came on fast. Weeks of agitation and nausea and a need to keep moving that reminded me of the akathisia but less extreme. Nights in bed with my heart thumping in my ears, not able to sleep, feeling adrenaline rushes through my chest.

The writing in my journal from that time doesn't seem like my own. The letters are lopsided but not in a scribble; the slant and indentation are too severe, the result of my fingers pressing the pen hard against the page. The words grasp at positivity. I write the same thing over and over: *I'm grateful for* ___ and fill in the blank with anything I can come up with. *I'm grateful for . . . those flowers . . . that lamp . . . my legs . . . the color of my eyes.*

The dates of the entries are scattered, and I wonder what happened in between. Some days must have been so bad they consisted of calling my sister and her directing me through our emergency plan: *benzo, CBT worksheet, sleep.* (Much the way *medications* had become *meds, benzodiazepines* had become *benzos*.) Succumb to unconsciousness. Wake and wish the symptoms of withdrawal would be gone: the cold sweats, the vertigo, the shaking, the diarrhea. Worst of all was the inability to focus my gaze, even with my glasses on, and the sense that the ground was undulating beneath me.

As I came off the antipsychotic and then the lithium, Dr. R was professional in the best sense of the word. He returned my calls the same day, always with an idea of what to do next. Sometimes, it was like listening to a witch brew a potion: a dab of Benadryl, a dash of the benzo, a hint more of the antipsychotic—for now.

The suicidality returned over Christmas break. Maybe it had to do with not teaching, not having anything to lift me out of it, even just for a few hours. One night, I sat on the edge of my bed, the phone pressed to my ear. My plan was clear: pills, a bottle of vodka, the tub. Through the phone came my sister's voice, not stern but strong and commanding. She'd become my lifeline, now that my mother was tending to her own emotional needs—and rightly so.

My sister asked, "Did you already take it?" *It* meaning the *benzo*.

"I don't want to," I said, tired of pills.

My sister is one of those rare people who can handle anything. She seems to know what to say or whom to call or where to go. When she says to do something, she's almost always right. "Go take it."

After I did and came back on the line, we went through the rest of my emergency plan. She walked me through a thought record, the CBT worksheet I held on to, which had me write down my thoughts and evaluate them, until the benzo knocked me out.

She asked if I wanted her to wait until I fell asleep.

"It's okay," I said.

"Are you sure?" she asked.

I nodded, a gesture she couldn't see. "Yes."

After we hung up, I crawled into bed, fully clothed.

13

On Solitude (and Isolation and Loneliness [and Brackets])

Even by studio standards, my apartment was tiny—the kitchen too close to the bed, the bed practically touching the bookshelf and the desk. It had a slight view of the Chicago skyline but mainly looked onto a brick wall. My immediate neighbors kept to themselves. They were presences, a series of doors opening and closing.

The suicidality eventually went away and the withdrawal symptoms stopped, only to be replaced by bone-deep anguish. I could barely be around people, even strangers on the street. By the time my meds were back to what they'd been with Dr. H—including the SSRI plus the benzo—I started to feel better and then well.

I had my mind back and could think clearly. I read—a lot. I thought—a lot. (Not pathological rumination; contemplation. [Though maybe too much.]) The only topic I avoided (except when I had to see Dr. R [and even then, I never asked which diagnosis he saw in me]) was mental illness. I existed like that for some time—in solitude.

The ideal of solitude is strength. It's a skill to be mastered: the ability to be alone without feeling lonely. It's decidedly male and often nationalistic, a symbol of American independence. It's Thoreau, who writes in *Walden* that he never felt lonesome "or in the least oppressed by a sense of solitude," except once, for an hour, when he "doubted if the near neighborhood of man was not essential to a serene and healthy life." (Of course, he may have found "the fancied advantages of human neighborhood insignificant" because his "solitary" cabin was on land owned by Emerson, his close neighbor. Thoreau often went to the Emersons' for dinner. He also entertained friends at his cabin and had his meals brought to him by his mother. That said, his Walden Pond experiment was less about living alone than living simply in nature.)

Solitude is righteous. It's Benjamin Rush—that controversial Founding Father who's often referred to as "the father of American psychiatry." Rush is credited for having saved people with mental illnesses from being seen as having been possessed by demons but also for subjecting them to bloodlettings and other gothic treatments. He considered solitude "among the physical causes which influence the moral faculty" for the better.

It's a source of wisdom. It's the Buddha on the path to enlightenment, Jesus and Moses in the desert, Muhammad on the mountain. It's Thomas Merton abandoning the vacuous debaucheries of New York City for the Trappist Abbey of Gethsemani. As he writes in *Thoughts in Solitude*, "When society is made of men who know no interior solitude it can no longer be held together by love: and consequently it is held together by a violent and abusive authority." For Merton, "interior solitude" is essential.

I never thought of myself as a recluse. True, I fit the secondary meaning of the word: a person removed from society. But the primary definition is one who retreats for religious reasons, and I didn't follow a faith. Besides, *recluse* has an air of eccentricity about it. It's J. D. Salinger (number one on *TIME* magazine's Top 10 Most Reclusive Celebrities list), forsaking publishing and granting a single interview every twenty or thirty years. It's Howard Hughes (number two on the list), who holed himself up in the Beverly Hills Hotel and let his fingernails and toenails grow—though, in all fairness, some speculate he may have suffered from a condition that made his nails both painful and difficult to clip. I wasn't a hermit either, which has a stronger religious connotation.

That time might best be described as urban solitude. I resided among people, passing them on the street, but never engaged. Not once did I dine out or go to the movies or to a museum. I taught—twelve hours a week, thirty weeks of the year, teaching at the same two universities, which, admittedly, offered a strong dose of social interaction. Teaching, mentoring, helping fulfilled me in a way nothing else did. Teaching gave me a dose of social interaction that could carry me for days. I worked out at a gym. I visited with my mother. But that was pretty much it. I saw no friends and rarely talked on the phone, even breaking off a friendship with someone dear to me who lived in another city and wanted to speak once a week to stay connected, because that much contact was unaccountably burdensome.

I didn't have an agoraphobic aversion to going out. My dislike of crowded places was reasonable: music festivals; parades; my nearby farmer's market, where people gathered to buy overpriced organic blueberries and artisan pizzas and to participate in drum circles. True, I avoided stores. Still, I existed in the world; I just happened to spend most of that existence in a one-room apartment.

I even had two weekslong relationships (or monthlong [though they were really a scattering of days]). It's hard to call them relationships. Both men lived in other cities, so I didn't see them more than a handful of times. Both had been in my life, years earlier, as friends. Both were solitaries, too. One lived on a remote farm in Michigan, the other in Portland, Oregon. Both went about their lives much the way I went about mine, albeit in larger spaces. (Both owned houses. No brick walls blocking their views.) Most of our interactions happened by text, which gives a false sense of intimacy. Frequent texting, with its vibrating interruptions into what might be an otherwise dull day, makes us feel wanted and attracted. But solitaries, I realized too late, don't do well together. There was a prickliness to us. A certain distance had to be maintained. Both relationships ended fiercely and fast, as if each of us had reached our saturation points of closeness and had to retreat or risk losing the edges—those brackets—that protected us.

My solitary walks followed the same route: under the bridge, north along the lagoon, past the driving range, to the harbor, and back. The park, which had once felt secluded, became downright desolate that winter. I didn't commune with the patches of nature portioned out to us in the city, barely noticing the red-winged blackbirds and the monarch butterflies or that an entire row of trees had died as a result of a beetle infestation and been cut down. The repetition and orderliness of following the same path was like a companion. There and back. There and back. In terms of traditional companionship, I was still inside myself. Blocked off.

Did my audiobooks count as companionship? No research has been done but studies show that hearing loss increases feelings of loneliness, so it would follow that the sound of another's voice in our ears—the gift of Toni Morrison reading *Beloved* or Gabriel Woolf reading *The Brothers Karamazov*—must do something for us.

Television and radio are considered companionship, though they're a slippery slope. According to researchers, watching a favorite show staves off loneliness, but a Netflix binge is a sign of it. Watching one episode functions as "social surrogacy" but sitting on the couch for ten hours to consume an entire season is a red flag. Radio, according to surveys conducted by media strategists and the BBC, can be a "lifeline." I watched a bit of television, mostly Nordic noir—*Forbrydelsen* and *Borgen* and *Bron/Broen*—but didn't listen to the radio.

And books. Research has shown that reading can contribute to feelings of connection and belonging but nothing has been studied specifically in terms of loneliness or isolation. My reading selections were odd. I read all of Patricia Highsmith's work. Highsmith was also a solitary who spent most of her life among snails and cats, both of which she apparently adored. She was a misanthrope and an alcoholic. In her stories and novels, she favors degenerate, predatory protagonists who cheat and steal and lie and murder and whom we end up rooting for. I reread *Strangers on a Train* so many times I lost count. It's fitting that I would immerse myself in a book about a seemingly fleeting human interaction so potent and dangerous that it gives one character enough power over the other to convince him to commit murder.

Social media didn't affect me very much. My followers on Twitter were barely in the double digits. I had hundreds and hundreds of friends on Facebook whom I didn't know, even by name. I didn't have an Instagram account. (How many arty, abstract photos of my brick wall could I post?) Many blame social media for America's collective loneliness, but studies don't support that view. One study found that only negative experiences on social media contribute to loneliness. Another reported social media can contribute to feelings of isolation but couldn't state definitively which came first: the isolation or social media. On the Cigna U.S. Loneliness Index, people who consistently used social media scored 44 percent whereas people who never used it scored 42 percent. It was a draw. In a Pew Research Center report, 81 percent of teens reported that social media enhances their friendships and 68 percent said they felt more supported by their friends because of it. In combating loneliness, the Cigna study shows that social media is less a factor than the quality of our interactions. Simply having people in our lives does little to assuage loneliness. One in four Americans feels misunderstood, two in five don't think their relationships are meaningful, and only half report having meaningful interactions daily.

––––––

Many people—scientists, psychologists, journalists, bloggers—distinguish between solitude and isolation. The binary is simplistic: solitude, good; isolation, bad. By definition, solitude and isolation are more nuanced than the good-bad binary makes them out to be. Solitude isn't all purity and fortitude. By definition, it's merely "the quality or state of being alone or remote from society" and can be "a lonely place." Isolation isn't necessarily punitive. The verb "to isolate" denotes the voluntary act of separating from others. It's benign, even positive: "occurring alone or once." Yet isolation is seen as a punishment, thrust upon us and never entered into by choice. The word connotes solitary confinement and incarceration—two tactics rooted in prejudice. The common remark that someone with a peaceful mind can enjoy isolation as monkish solitude whereas someone with a troubled mind will suffer solitude as imprisonment misses the fact that a monk typically isn't in a forty-eight-square-foot cell, could not possibly have been arrested as a result of racial profiling, and is free to leave at any time.

I could leave but never went far. No vacation. No quick road trip out of the city. I rarely went outside a five-mile radius. Same bed. Same breakfast, lunch, and dinner table. Same desk. Same walls.

———

My apartment stopped suiting me. It wasn't a refuge anymore. No relief came at being alone each time I walked through the door. That small space no longer provided solitude. Solitude slid into isolation and isolation tipped over into loneliness. I blamed the claustrophobic lack of square footage, the oppressive brick wall. Even before I walked in the door, I felt a crushing weight.

The essayist Michel de Montaigne would have disagreed. Physical space doesn't determine our emotions; the mind does: "Our disease lies in the mind, which cannot escape from itself." Montaigne would have told me to keep a "back shop," a private room within the self, where others can't enter. Plaster and wood have nothing to do with it. We must have "a mind pliable in itself, that will be company." Finding contentment in solitude requires self-reliance. But my inner back shop had transformed from a citadel of solitude to a penitentiary of isolation and loneliness.

Like the solitude-good, isolation-bad calculation, a similar binary is applied to solitude and loneliness, except loneliness isn't just bad, it's dangerous. In the US, it's an "epidemic" that affects teenagers and the elderly most acutely. It's a health threat on par with smoking, contributing to heart disease and increasing the risk of stroke, Type 2 diabetes, dementia, and suicide. Loneliness affects how we work, making us less likely to succeed and take pleasure in what we do.

But loneliness isn't threatening. It means "being without company." Only the tertiary and quaternary definitions emotionalize it as "sad from being alone" and "producing a feeling of bleakness or desolation."

Loneliness, like any difficult emotion, gets its power from the conviction that we're the only ones feeling it. As a defense, we reassure ourselves that others feel it, too. We join loneliness meetup groups and form people-haters clubs. Thousands of us like the books cited on the loneliness-quotes page on Goodreads. Eleven thousand people liked a passage from Jodi Picoult's bestseller *My Sister's Keeper*: "Let me tell you this: if you meet a loner, no matter what they tell you, it's not because they enjoy solitude. It's because they have tried to blend into the world before, and people continue to disappoint them." The loner, the lonely one, isn't to blame; it's other people.

Discomfort is, by nature, uncomfortable. Days spent in my apartment were jarring. Even my solitary walks became unnerving. But I didn't call my discomfort *symptoms*.

———

The change didn't come as a chrysalis moment. Not an instant of blossoming. It came as a slow unraveling facilitated in part by a book. I entered my pathological life through one book—*The Best Little Girl in the World*—and exited it through another—the DSM.

It's unclear why I suddenly wanted to know the source of my diagnosis. Maybe it was the solitude. Or the discomfort. My doctoral program taught me to rely on primary sources. I hadn't been doing that.

I wish I could say my first real encounter with the DSM took place in the dim, dusty stacks of a medical library, but I was in my tiny apartment in the blue light of my computer screen. My desk lamp was lit. A half-nibbled square of chocolate sat on a paper towel beside my keyboard. An internet window was open to the library portal of the university where I taught. I typed *DSM* in the search box and filtered for online access: *Diagnostic and Statistical Manual of Mental Disorders: DSM-5. American Psychiatric Association. DSM-5 Task Force. c2013.*

I clicked and scrolled past the purple cover to the introduction. The sense that, if I kept reading, it might contaminate me and I might somehow fall back into that world of diagnoses and Dr. Ms and PHPs almost made me stop. But I clicked on the *Bipolar and Related Disorders* chapter. It was all there: short paragraphs describing each disorder followed by numbered and alphabetical symptoms lists followed by codes and specifiers and "diagnostic features."

People complain that these lists and categories are what's wrong with the DSM. But to me they were beautiful. Clear. Orderly.

Then I found other books warning against accepting DSM diagnoses. In *Saving Normal: An Insider's Revolt against Out-of-Control Psychiatric Diagnosis, DSM-5, Big Pharma, and the Medicalization of Ordinary Life*, Allen Frances writes, "[New] diagnoses in psychiatry are potentially much more dangerous than new drugs because they can lead to massive overtreatment (with all the possible side effects)."[1] In *The Loss of Sadness: How Psychiatry Transformed Normal Sorrow into Depressive Disorder* by Allan Horwitz and Jerome Wakefield, they state: "Pathologization of normal conditions may cause harm, and avoidance of such pathologization may decrease such harm."[2] I read Edward Shorter's *A History of Psychiatry* and *How Everyone Became Depressed: The Rise and Fall of the Nervous Breakdown*. And Hannah Decker's *The Making of DSM-III: A Diagnostic Manual's Conquest of American Psychiatry*. And Anne Harrington's *Mind Fixers: Psychiatry's Troubled Search for the Biology of Mental Illness*. And Thomas Szasz. And Robert Whitaker. And Erving Goffman.

And *The Book of Woe*, in which Gary Greenberg eviscerates the DSM. He asks psychiatry for one—just one—"slam dunk" diagnosis: "the psychiatric equivalent of strep or diabetes, a single diagnosis that indicated a single pathology and a single treatment. But I would have settled for less, one solid example of the value of a diagnostic system."[3] Spoiler: He never finds one.

The truth was everywhere but nowhere. Most people I knew still believed in the chemical imbalance theory. They talked about their "depression" and "anxiety disorder" as actual illnesses and took medication and saw psychiatrists and psychologists and therapists (though how many would if they didn't have insurance and had to pay out of pocket?), all without knowing what the acronym DSM even stood for. The truth was in plain sight (but hidden [bracketed]).

———

Another chrysalis moment came in late January. A kind of cracking. Different: outer shell cracking.

The wind whistled through the unsealed gaps in my windows. I woke and pulled up the shades to find them covered in frost, making it hard to see outside. I couldn't even glimpse the brick wall. The weather app showed a "feels like" temperature of negative 40 degrees Fahrenheit. A Google search revealed that a public-health advisory had been issued, warning people to stay inside. Schools and businesses were closed.

Before the change, this would have been just another day in my apartment. I ate breakfast, wrote for a while, and graded papers. I'd finished washing my spoon and cereal bowl when my skin started to itch. I scratched my forearms, inciting the itch. Soon my skin was red and puffy. I put Cortaid on it, and the itching dissipated a bit.

Back at my desk, sitting at the computer, the shades drawn to keep out the cold, my dark felt oppressively small. The walls didn't close in but I became increasingly aware of their closeness.

I tugged at my turtleneck. My mouth went dry. I couldn't swallow. My only thought was *Out*.

None of my neighbors were in the hallway. No one joined me in the elevator. The lobby, too, was vacant.

I stood at the glass-door entrance of my building, which wasn't covered in frost, and peered out at what might have been a portrait of extinction. No cars passed on the street, no pedestrians on the sidewalk. Whereas once being cut off wouldn't have fazed me, a wave of isolation and loneliness crashed over me. I saw in my reflection a woman very much alone but ready to reach out.

That force, that reaching, was more powerful than the one that had pulled me into myself. It propelled me out. The propelling wasn't pleasant. My whole default mode ruptured. I felt exposed, my brick walls and frosted windows demolished. My life was no longer bracketed in the same way.

———

The next morning, I called my sister. Her voice had the measured tone of someone ready for a crisis. No crisis, I said, and asked if I could work at her house that day.

She set me up in their living room on their L-shaped couch and there I stayed and worked as they went about their lives: my nephew leaving for tennis practice, my brother-in-law coming home from work, my niece down in the basement (under the stairs in a kind of fort she built [a spot she loved]) doing her homework, my sister caring for all of us. My niece and nephew, who were too young to be told what was happening, never questioned why I was over so much. Their ordinary hellos were a balm. My brother-in-law, too, wore a facial expression that always seemed to say, *Here if you need me.*

With one call, I could invoke the kind of social support few have. In my IOPs, during group therapy sessions, more often than not someone spoke about how their families didn't understand. As we sat in a circle and listened to each other, one woman, tears in her eyes, her legs crossed, her long dark hair falling in front of her face, said that her sister, having found out about her diagnosis, would no longer let her babysit her niece. I always knew my sister, my mother, my father, my stepmother, my brother-in-law, my niece and nephew were there for me.

———

Over the next few months, I settled into new patterns. A reasonable part of my day was spent in the company of others—family, acquaintances, colleagues, strangers. I didn't just notice people; I took note of them: the cashier at the grocery store, the person behind me in line, the Uber driver, the couple at a nearby table. Each day, upon returning to my building, I rode the elevator and stood in silence with my neighbors. Most of them stared down at their phones. When we reached my floor, I wished them a good evening, smiled, and tried to make eye contact with at least one person. Some responded with surprise, others like I'd startled them. One guy furrowed his brow with annoyance, almost offense, as if I'd invaded his personal space (or solitude [or isolation (or loneliness [as if I'd trespassed his brackets])]). Some made eye contact and wished me the same. Others responded with a mechanical "You, too," without glancing up from their phones.

At first, their responses mattered, but I realized that wasn't the point. The key to connection was not to be needy of connection with others. We have to give freely of ourselves, act as social philanthropists who donate anonymously, expecting no plaques or appreciation in return.

It didn't take meaningful interactions to infiltrate my isolation, curb my loneliness, and spur my recovery. Noticing other people was enough. My "have a good evening" and "have a good one" communications provided "meaningful interaction."

What constitutes "meaningful interaction"? What degree of intimacy does it require? What emotions do we need to experience before, during, and after for it to qualify? Holding people to such high standards (or any standards) seems to invite feelings of isolation and loneliness.

Which isn't to say I didn't feel isolated or lonely or struggle not to feel unwell; I did. Returning to my apartment still filled me with dread, especially in the winter, when I was met by late-afternoon darkness. Loneliness seemed to wait by the door to welcome me home. The sickening black mass in my stomach came and went. But the feelings and sensations passed in a way they hadn't before.

––––––

The time I spent in solitude (or isolation [or loneliness]) is bracketed; that's how it's punctuated for me now. Inside it are the changing cocktail of medications, the withdrawal symptoms, the suicidality, the nausea, Dr. M, the PHPs. Over. Tucked away. Inside each other.

One night when I was teaching ESL at the community center in Brooklyn, I double-checked the answer to a grammar question about parentheses. The students worked in pairs, parsing workbook exercises in English—such a difficult language with its changing grammar rules and high-maintenance punctuation marks. I opened my copy of *Warriner's English Grammar and Composition* to the page on brackets.

Brackets signify a double enclosure in a text. They're commonly used in citations but can also indicate parenthetical thoughts. Thoughts inside thoughts: *(I am solitary [or am I isolated?].)* They illustrate the way the mind works (most minds [or perhaps only my mind]), with its reservations and clarifications and contradictions. One thought can be a statement, another a question. One can communicate certainty, another doubt. Though some grammarians say that brackets include unnecessary information, this is far from true: Brackets represent our internal lives, our deepest secrets.

Rarely do we use brackets this way—most grammarians would opt for commas or dashes—but brackets occupy the primary position on two keys on the QWERTY keyboard while parentheses (which we use more often) are relegated to secondary positions above the nine and the zero. Maybe we don't communicate through brackets to avoid experiencing the depths of ourselves. If commas are speed bumps, dashes open doors, and parentheses are hurdles to step over, then brackets are solid walls.

The origins of brackets—once referred to as crotchets—are shrouded in mystery (pun intended). A sibling of parentheses [( )] and chevrons (< >), brackets are said to have been invented at the turn of the fourteenth century by the Italian humanist and rhetorician Coluccio Salutati.[4] Editors often used them to make comments and corrections on a text. In a twist of imagination, they show up in Samuel Richardson's 1748 epistolary novel *Clarissa* (a tome I've actually read) and in Laurence Sterne's 1759 novel *Tristram Shandy* (a tome I haven't) to express material omitted not by the editor or the author, which would later become common, but by the characters.

Like marks of parentheses, brackets might be seen as broken pieces of what once was whole. Parentheses appear as a circle divided in two:

O ( )

Brackets are a broken square:

$$\square \quad [\ ]$$

They emit a feeling of enclosure. Which is how I see myself during those years: walled off, the self alone with the self, inside the self.

Brackets, like human beings, are relational. At times they signal unnecessary information; at others, they draw attention to what's inside. Recently, someone reminded me that they hold space [ ] for words that may or may not yet exist. They communicate to the reader when someone's words have been altered. In quotations, they show when only part of a sentence is being quoted but presented as a stand-alone clause: *It's possible she has depression* becomes *[S]he has depression.* It can tell us when someone else's words have been manipulated, a boundary has been inserted to connect two voices, perhaps causing the meaning to change. Brackets clarify the context: *She has an illness [bipolar].* They nest information: *She has an illness (bipolar [which she's been told is lifelong]).* They point out a typo or an error in the original text: *She's really bipolr [sic].* Not my error; someone else's.

―――――

"Listen," Dr. R said, holding up his hands, signaling me to wait. "It isn't always clear."

We were in his office in our respective leather chairs. I'd asked what he thought was my diagnosis.

He gave me one.

I nodded, though not in agreement. His diagnosis was *his* diagnosis—the DSM's diagnosis. How could I accept what wasn't valid?

We made a follow-up appointment. I walked down the long hallway and rode the elevator to the lobby. The almost-spring air outside was moist and cool. A last-bit-of-winter wind blew down Chicago Avenue. Patches of ice melted on the sidewalk.

14

On Stigma (and Disclosure)

One morning, I woke with a moan—an audible moan: dark, bellowing, but not so loud that the neighbors would hear. I emailed my editor and then opened the blinds covering my window. It was oppressively sunny. Even the blue sky seemed wrong.

It started the day before. A friend and I sat eating turkey sandwiches in the seating area of Whole Foods. She knew some of what I'd been through. I mentioned that I was going on the academic job market. She worked in human resources.

I said, "I'm a little worried about—"

"Oh, don't be. The stigma against mental illness—" She glanced around and lowered her voice. "It's so much better now."

"No, I'm worried about someone seeing this." On my phone, I pulled up an essay I'd published about one of my suicidal episodes. It had seemed like a good idea: writing as therapy, helping others by telling my story. But it was the first piece that came up in a Google search of my name. I imagined members of a hiring committee scrolling through the essay. It seemed as if I had to ask the magazine to take it down from their site.

She looked down at the screen. She didn't read far before she said, "Yeah, maybe it's not a good idea to have that out there."

Back in my office, I thought, *No.* Wasn't academia the upholder of open-mindedness? Didn't I work in "the humanities"? Didn't universities post in their job descriptions equal opportunities for people who "have or have had" a mental illness?

A colleague read the essay. We sat in her office. "You cannot take this down," she said and spoke of artistic freedom. When I asked what a hiring committee's response might be, she hesitated. "Maybe leave it off your CV and *don't* include it in your writing sample."

Another colleague read it. His expression clouded with concern. Definitely leave it off my CV, definitely don't include it in my writing sample, probably take it off the site.

———

Stigma (which literally means a branding with a hot iron on the skin and figuratively a mark of disgrace) against suicide plays out in stereotypes, discrimination, and the prejudice that it's the act of someone with an unhinged mind. The nature of the stigma differs across genders, races, cultures, and socioeconomic classes, but it affects us all.[1] It's done nothing to decrease suicide rates, which have increased over the past twenty years.[2]

Historically, suicide has been portrayed as weak, sacrilegious, a mortal sin, evil, demonic, criminal, selfish, egotistical, and the sign of a deranged mind. Saint Augustine was the first to twist scripture and denounce self-murder as a sin. In the fourth century, he condemned it based on his interpretation of the fifth commandment. In his *Confessions*, he wrote, "God's command 'Thou shalt not kill' is to be taken as forbidding self-destruction."

The idea that it was somehow a marker of insanity came from Elizabethan England. The only way to avoid being posthumously charged with self-murder was to be deemed non compos mentis, otherwise you'd be denied a Christian burial, have your body thrown naked into the ground, be skewered with a wooden stake, and have your family punished and impoverished. The suicide of a "lunatic" was accepted because it was to be expected, given their mental state.

The DSM stigmatizes suicide. In the DSM-IV, suicidality was

considered either a symptom or complication of certain diagnoses, particularly mood disorders and substance abuse disorders. The DSM-5 proposed *suicidal behavior disorder* (SBD), which could be diagnosed in anyone who had attempted suicide any time in the past twenty-four months.[3] *Twenty-four months.* Two years. That means that someone who has tried to end her life and survived a mental struggle the intensity of which few can fathom can continue to be labeled "mentally ill" for as long as two years, one-fifth of a decade. That's not a diagnosis, not treatment; that's condemnation and punishment. A sentence greater than many actual crimes. In my home state of Illinois, aggravated assault—a felony, depending on the circumstances—can get less than a year.[4]

I'd never champion suicide—no one should have to experience a doubt that vicious—but it hasn't always been denounced as an act against God, nature, the state, the community, one's family, and oneself. Likewise, it has not always been treated as evidence of an unstable mind—not to the Stoics in Ancient Greece,[5] not to the Ancient Romans,[6] and not to Shakespeare, who often depicted suicides in his plays sympathetically.[7] Not to many Enlightenment thinkers like David Hume, who practically argued in favor of it—mainly from his position as a rationalist in favor of personal freedom and against religious dogma.[8] Not to African American slaves, who saw it as an act of resistance and even power.[9] Not to Émile Durkheim, who saw it as more a result of cultural and social factors than an individual's disposition or choice.[10] Not to the French theorist Michel Foucault, who believed it to be a reasonable, deviant act censured unfairly by those in power.[11]

Still, I had good reason to believe I should take down the essay and hide it. The stigma was real. Mental illness and DSM diagnoses were one thing, but suicide was . . . extreme. It crossed a line. What would my niece and nephew think if they knew? Who would want to be in a relationship with someone who'd wanted to end her life? How could a committee privy to that information hire me, given how competitive the market was, flooded with writers and PhDs who wouldn't (this was the assumption) cause them problems?

———

When my editor's response finally arrived in my in-box, it was too long to be a simple *Yes, right away*. She said she understood my concerns, but the piece, she wrote, had been getting a lot of traffic. This wasn't meant in a more-hits-for-the-magazine way; it was reaching and helping people. And then there was the artist who'd done the artwork to consider. In many ways, the essay had become a collective effort and was no longer mine to take down. She asked me to think about it.

At my appointment with Dr. R that day, I asked what he thought. He settled back in his plush leather chair and crossed his legs in a figure four. His eyes widened. He grimaced as if to say, *Tough one*.

"To some degree," he said, his chin bobbing in the affirmative, "you should keep your mental health history private. So no. In most professional environments and especially in academia, people don't understand." He smiled that strange smile and shook his head. "Now, if you were applying to law school or med school, I'd say go for it. They love that shit."

That night, in the blue of my laptop screen, I read my essay online again. I caught some mistakes and didn't agree with some of it. It seemed to have been written by someone else. How could someone write something like that? How could she talk about suicide so openly?

I went to the window. The brick wall stared back at me. No one would hire someone who was once suicidal, who once knew the semicolon firsthand. More thoughts came. I had to hide the essay.

———

In her next email, my editor told me it wasn't the magazine's policy to take published work off the site and offered to use only my first name and last initial and remove my bio so no one would recognize me. In a few weeks, she said, Google's algorithm would work its magic, and no one would be able to link me to the essay again.

I went for a walk through the park. The overcast sky was low to the ground. A thin fog made the red and yellow autumn leaves glisten. I should have felt unburdened, but my chest became heavy. I'd abandoned the essay and was pretending it wasn't mine. I felt empty: no diagnosis, no answer, no past.

But I did have a past. On a similar afternoon the year before, I'd walked that same route. Same overcast sky though no fog. Same leaves. Same trees. Same tree I'd wanted to hang myself from.

Maybe taking my name off the essay (pretending it wasn't mine) was a wise way to control my life's narrative. Not that it would work. Each emergency room visit was on my medical record. My suicidal ideations could be found in Dr. C's and Dr. H's and Dr. M's notes. My six diagnoses, too, were permanent. Each had its own set of consequences. Bipolar alone would make it hard for me to adopt a child. Life insurance would be difficult to get.

Back at my apartment, I pulled up the web page with my essay: "On Suicidal Ideation" by Sarah F. *Sarah F.* So close to anonymous. It wasn't me. It was the right thing to do—the only thing I could do. No one needed to know.

———

At my next appointment with Dr. R, I told him I wanted off all my meds. He'd changed my diagnosis—for the third time. I'd decided to live without one. If I wasn't going to accept a diagnosis and was going to hide my past, I couldn't be on meds. That wouldn't make sense.

Dr. R crossed his legs in a figure four and settled back in his chair. "I had a client—worst diagnosis you can have: schizoaffective disorder. I mean, bipolar topped with schizophrenia? Can't get worse than that. She was from a family of litigators—*famous* litigators. *Not* what a psychiatrist wants. I told her family what we needed to do. Her family informed me of what *they* thought we needed to do. As far as I knew, they didn't have a medical degree among them. But I said, 'Fine, take her to Mass General, best in the country for this sort of thing, and get a second opinion.' They flew her out to Boston on their private plane.

The docs at Mass General disagreed with me. Fine. Six weeks after her treatment started at Mass General, their daughter was *worse*. The family came back to me. We did what I'd said. It took time, but she got better. Once she was better, she said she wanted off the drugs. Fine. Slowly, we took her off them. *Slowly*. She's now an executive at Google. Off all meds."

"That's what I want," I said.

He looked away. On his face was an expression of *that's not going to happen* or maybe *that wasn't the point of the story*. He suggested we raise the dose of my SSRI.

"Why?" I asked, my voice cracking. I'd managed to get off the antipsychotic and the lithium and quit the benzo (in one day—I still hadn't known the dangers), so why not the SSRI and the lamotrigine?

"It's not worth it," he said. "Those medications aren't hurting you. Low-side-effect profiles."

I said I was determined.

He uncrossed his legs and breathed deeply. "Okay, we can try with the lamotrigine."

I became enamored with "the withdrawal community." Made up of laypeople with no medical training, it encouraged people to get off their meds. The media had embraced it. A *New York Times* article on psychiatric drug withdrawal portrayed those going off psychiatric drugs as heroes struggling to overcome great odds and winning.[12] The *New Yorker* ran a profile about (really a paean to) one withdrawal community leader, praising her for stopping her medications without medical supervision, becoming free, and encouraging others (and charging money to advise them) to do the same.[13] To be medication-free was to be mentally pure and psychopharmacologically virtuous.

The withdrawal community was pill-shaming me, and I believed they were right. They preached the necessity of breaking free of psychotropic drugs without relying on my doctor's help. One site wrote I was "the only person who can decide if and how [I'll] taper off." Before I could enter the site, I had to click a box absolving them of responsibility for anything that happened as a result of reading such statements. I empathized with a blogger who wrote her doctor told her that if she really wanted off her meds, she'd just stop. Another blogger quipped that not getting off my medications was "giving up." Another encouraged me to "keep going," so I did.

––––––

Physicians, researchers, and academics battle in print and on TV and on podcasts and at podiums as to whether psychotropic drugs save people or destroy them.[14] The pro-medication side tends to be made up of psychiatrists, academics, and researchers with conflicts of interest so deep the studies read as Big Pharma pamphlets. The con/deprescribe-now side includes disgruntled psychiatrists and psychiatric survivors who tend to demonize psychiatric medications.[15]

The deprescribe-now-ers inadvertently scared me into wanting off my meds. Robert Whitaker's *Mad in America* podcast spoke of the dangers of psychopharmacology: the wonder drugs and "breakthrough" medications that reinforced diagnoses; the billions made by drug companies; the exclusively short-term benefits of psychiatric medications; and the toxic, dangerous long-term effects. Patient-advocate psychiatrist Peter Breggin said psychiatric drugs were toxins and didn't cure mental illnesses; they were the reason for them: "[T]hey aren't correcting biochemical imbalances, they are causing biochemical imbalances."[16] Whitaker, Breggin, and others convincingly argued that antipsychotics and antianxiety medications actually produced psychosis and anxiety.[17]

––––––

A week later, I stood behind the podium teaching my Introduction to Literature course. We were discussing Amy Tan's essay "Mother Tongue." In it, Tan tells of the discrimination her mother faced because she speaks what Tan calls "broken English"—a mix of English and Chinese grammar, punctuation, and syntax; words put together with comma splices and without verbs. A student said that the point of the essay wasn't about "like, speaking, like, perfect English" but to appreciate bilingualism.

I started to sweat. My heart raced. More sweating.

A student raised his hand and shared that he was the child of first-generation immigrants and had had the same experience with his parents.

Soon, sweat had soaked my bra, my camisole, my shirt, and was starting to go through my blazer. Luckily, my blazer was black, so my students couldn't see.

After class, in my office, I draped my clothes on my bookshelf to dry. Dr. R had assured me that going off the lamotrigine caused no withdrawal symptoms. I called and left him a message.

When he returned my call, I said I couldn't go through it again.

He reassured me—genuinely—that it was okay. We'd hit on the lowest dosage I could stand. He told me to go back up on the lamotrigine to where we were.

Maybe it was okay. Maybe DSM diagnoses could be fictitious without it meaning that medications don't help some people. Drug studies are based on false DSM diagnoses. They test using the DSM's random symptom lists, using as subjects people they can't prove have the same disorder—or any disorder.

But maybe I could reject the DSM's diagnoses and still have or have had a mental illness and continue to be on medication. Maybe I didn't have to embrace or reject the mental health industrial complex entirely. Maybe I could live without clarity or symptom lists or order or an answer. If I did, I had to accept my suicidality and pull it from the parentheses.

———

Parentheses typify interiority and withholding. They date back to before the Renaissance.[18] In the sixteenth century, the Dutch philosopher and scholar Desiderius Erasmus called them *lunulae*, little moons. One of their earliest uses was by the Elizabethan rhetorician, scholar, and scribe Angel Day. As a scribe, Day would have been privy to and trusted with his employer's secrets. Parentheses might be seen as a closed circle, a covenant, divided in two:

O ( )

The *Oxford English Dictionary* would later define them as "an explanation, aside, or afterthought" without grammatical relevance to the rest of the sentence. Often, parenthetical punctuation marks—parentheses, dashes, and commas—are described as interchangeable. But parentheses couldn't be more different from dashes or parenthetical commas. Parentheses (at first) seem prohibitive. They take effort to get into. They stop us only to whisper an invitation for us to climb inside. They're inner thoughts and secrets.

———

At my next appointment, I asked Dr. R about the long-term side effects of the drugs I was on. He looked out the window and paused. "According to the literature—I mean, what we know now; it's unlikely. You mean now? There are some data...What we know now? No, there are no serious risks."

I could have tried to find meaning in his words, the stuttered phrases between the quotation marks; decoded every comma, each period, the dash and ellipsis, the semicolon, the apostrophe, the question mark, every space. I could have ruminated on them, inserting slashes of indecision—*believe this/that, accept the diagnosis/don't accept it*—but I didn't.

Epilogue

My new living room window gives me a view of the lake and the city skyline. The sun is rising, turning the horizon a deep pink hue. In the kitchen, on the counter—a new counter, this one speckled gray—sits my blue pillbox.

I pop the tab. No longer "meds," they're just pills I take. One gets stuck in my throat. The taste—tinny—lingers, even after I wash it down with water.

It's a luxury to refuse a diagnosis (or two or four or six), to refute the certainty presumed by the DSM. I'm not in crisis. My diagnosis wasn't forced on me as a method of social control. I don't need the diagnosis to receive disability payments. My pills work (though I don't know if they're needed to treat a condition or because my body is dependent on them). I found the right combination and dosage of medications, which is like finding the slimmest of needles in the largest of haystacks at the end of a rainbow after winning the lottery.

It would be different if I were transgender and needed my diagnosis to receive medical care. Sadly, according to the DSM, being transgender is a mental illness. Originally called sexual deviation, then a personality disorder, then a sexual and gender identity disorder, it's now known as "gender dysphoria." The authors of the DSM-5 insist the new label only applies to those in distress. That would be true if transgender people weren't forced to accept the diagnosis to get necessary treatments.

Some find power in their diagnoses. When Asperger's was removed from the DSM-5 and replaced with autism spectrum disorder, the outcry from the Asperger's community was thunderous. Aspies, as they call themselves, relish the label given to them. It's part of their identity, offering access to treatment and a sense of belonging.

But accepting the DSM's unsubstantiated diagnoses—believing them, applying them, becoming them—almost drove me to suicide. That time is filled with the joining of illogical thoughts using a comma (*He says I'm sick, so I must be sick*), lists of symptoms and side effects following a colon (*She shows many of the symptoms: inflated mood, depressive episodes, irritability*), hyphenated terms (*direct-to-consumer marketing*), unanswerable questions (*Am I really sick?*), points when I should have put a stop to things (*Enough.*) and given myself options (*bipolar/not bipolar*), alarm bells that should have sounded (*Don't listen!*) but didn't. Questions still come: *Had I made myself ill? Had I made it all up? Was it mental illness or the effects of medications? How much of it was me and how much others telling me I was sick? How can I be on medication but reject a diagnosis?* I have some answers: *no, no, uncertain, a lot, because I am.*

———

The power of suggestion may have played a role in how I became well. We're influenced by "experts." Jean-Martin Charcot "cured" patients suffering from hysteria using hypnosis. The neurologist George Beard acknowledged[1] the effect of expectation, which can[2] be positive or negative, depending on what we believe. Dr. R said he'd get me well—not medication-free but functioning, often high functioning, even whatever I imagine "Google-executive high functioning" to be.

But I never believed him to be the mythical genius/irreverent doctor so often found in the classic mental-illness memoir. He wasn't Sherman to my Kessa. He didn't make me well; my words to myself did. When I stopped labeling and talking to myself as a sick person, I no longer was one.

Not that I'm emotionally at ease. I *feel* depression and anxiety—sometimes deeply, paralyzingly—but I don't *have* depression or anxiety.

The stomachaches still come, as does the edginess, although I don't let it veer into splintering or cracking. No derealization or depersonalization but plenty of loneliness and isolation. And solitude. And hope.

Therapy never helped me understand myself better. Maybe I just didn't find the right therapist. My therapy sessions consisted of complaining and talking at length about situations and events that usually didn't deserve that much attention or that became a bigger deal by talking about them. They kept me in the past; I want to live into my future.

One thing did help me understand myself—or at least my mind and body—a little better: evolutionary psychiatry. Unsurprisingly, my exposure to that branch of psychiatry started with a book: physician and scientist Randolph Nesse's *Good Reasons for Bad Feelings: Insights from the Frontier of Evolutionary Psychiatry*. My father and I started having lunch together every Sunday. (It quickly became one of the highlights of my week.) I may have suggested we read Nesse's book, but most likely my father did. (It was one of *The Economist*'s "Books of the Year," and my father is devoted to *The Economist*.) Nesse offers a paradigm I'd never considered. Maybe emotions like anxiety and depression aren't pathological; maybe they date back to primitive humankind and for some reason haven't been eliminated by natural selection. Anxiety (even edginess) may have helped primitive humans stay alert and run from lions on the veldt. According to some theories, depression might be a reasonable—even evolutionarily beneficial—way of responding to stress.[3]

Nesse applies the methods of evolutionary biology to offer an alternative psychiatric approach to the DSM's symptom lists and tome of diagnoses. The mind is perfectly designed to respond to danger; the problem is that most people live comparatively free of threat. My often extreme emotions, responses, and thoughts are natural but no longer useful. They aren't necessarily a sign of disorder or disease. Sometimes painful emotions are necessary; sometimes they're not. The emotion of depression (a slowing, a weight) could be the body's response to extended periods of the emotion of anxiety (rushes of adrenaline, edginess, the sense of splintering and then cracking).

What I liked most about Nesse's book is his transparency. He presents theories, not "truths." Unlike the DSM's authors, he doesn't presume scientific authority where there is none. Evolutionary psychiatry isn't a treatment and has no ties to pharmaceutical companies. Nesse stresses that it offers only "philosophical insights."[4]

Evolutionary psychiatry isn't perfect, but its insights helped me view my mind differently. The mind isn't some evil entity full of repression and hidden nightmares and driven by sinister ulterior motives and meanings. It's not a series of uncontrollable chemical imbalances and stray synapses and wayward neurons. Certainly it's not the source of thoughts and behaviors that fall on symptom lists that qualify me for diagnoses in the DSM. It's a well-intended machine trying to keep me safe through worry, anxiety, dread, and depression.

Even my suicidality could be understood as a natural, albeit incorrect evolutionary response.[5] It wasn't sinful or shameful or evidence of "insanity." It wasn't driven by self-hatred. It was my primitive mind telling me that I was dependent on the collective to survive and that if I was a burden and no longer reproducing or of use, altruistic suicide was the answer. None of that was relevant to my life, and my suicidality wasn't altruistic, but the brain may be conditioned to that evolutionary paradigm and perhaps had mistakenly offered suicide as a viable option. This is a simplistic view, one that doesn't take into account the torment of suicidality, which is a descent to a dark, excruciating place no one should ever have to go, but it's also more generous and less stigmatizing than others.[6]

I reject a diagnosis because none has been proven, but I have or had a mental illness—broadly and without definition. I have certain limitations or, if that sounds too ableist, follow certain guidelines. My body and mind demand a level of care that many don't need. I live simply, modestly. Most would call my existence decidedly dull: healthy diet, little travel, lots of fresh air and exercise, no drugs, no alcohol, no caffeine, little sugar, routine schedule. I don't make these choices because I have a DSM diagnosis (or two or four or six) but to be well.

I'm not anti-psychiatry though there are plenty of reasons to be. Psychiatrists attend conferences at which their colleagues present data that support the use of psychiatric medications from research funded by the drug companies that produced those drugs. They fail to report their conflicts of interest.[7] They accept gifts and samples from drug reps and then present their patients with a veritable buffet of drugs to choose from.[8] Psychiatrists like Joseph Biederman, Charles Nemeroff, and Alan Schatzberg (the same Alan Schatzberg who passed off SSRI withdrawal as "discontinuation syndrome") accepted millions from drug companies or, in Schatzberg's case, held $4.8 million in stockholdings in the drug company he cofounded, which produced psychiatric medications he endorsed. Biederman "helped to fuel a fortyfold increase from 1994 to 2003 in the diagnosis of pediatric bipolar disorder" and proselytized the use of antipsychotics in children.[9] As the director of the Johnson & Johnson Center for Pediatric Psychopathology Research at Massachusetts General Hospital, he accepted kickbacks from and promised Johnson & Johnson—producer of the antipsychotic Risperdal, which was marketed to children with "pediatric bipolar disorder"—that his studies would support the safety and effectiveness of Risperdal, aiding sales.[10] Over his career, he accepted more than $1.6 million in "consulting fees" from drug companies while conducting clinical trials that produced favorable outcomes for antipsychotics marketed by those drug companies to children. After a congressional investigation, he wasn't fired from either of his prestigious positions at Harvard Medical School and Massachusetts General Hospital and continued to teach aspiring psychiatrists. He wasn't reprimanded for accepting the money, only for not reporting it.[11] There were few repercussions, the most severe being that he was prohibited from being paid by pharma for just one year and then "monitored" for just two years. Harvard saw "a delay of consideration for promotion or advancement" a suitable reparation, even though Biederman was already a full professor with the luxury of tenure.[12]

I'm not anti-medication even though the outrage against big pharma is wholly justified. Drug companies ply academic psychiatrists with gifts and fund their research and call them "key opinion leaders," which amounts to little more than paying them to promote their drugs. They get patients to diagnose and medicate themselves through ask-your-doctor campaigns. They create diagnoses and epidemics, as in 1998, when GlaxoSmithKline requested FDA approval for Paxil and hired the PR firm Cohn & Wolfe to market not the drug but generalized anxiety disorder (GAD), which soon reached "epidemic" proportions.[13]

The FDA allows off-label prescriptions, a multibillion-dollar industry. The government permits direct-to-consumer advertising. Mental health organizations take drug company money—including NAMI, which apparently between 1996 and mid-1999 took $11.72 million from Janssen ($2.08 million), Novartis ($1.87 million), Pfizer ($1.3 million), Abbott Laboratories ($1.24 million), Wyeth-Ayerst Pharmaceuticals ($658,000), Bristol Myers Squibb ($613,505), and Eli Lilly.[14] (One could argue that there's no conflict of interest when an organization like NAMI takes drug company money because it helps people with mental illnesses and people with mental illnesses take pharmaceutical drugs, but doing so creates suspicions of a quid pro quo relationship, especially when NAMI advises people to take said drugs.) The Depression Awareness, Recognition, and Treatment (DART) Program promoted by the National Institute of Mental Health was a team effort with drug companies to convince the public that depressive disorders were "common, serious" diseases treatable with medication.[15]

The anti-medication movement is, in many ways, misdirected and potentially harmful. No, we don't really know how psychiatric medications work and yes, most arose from unethical conditions and yes, they're overprescribed, but they help some of us and some desperately need any help available. Going off medication, particularly without a physician's care, as some in the withdrawal community advise, can be very, very dangerous.

Demonizing psychiatry and pill-shaming doesn't get at the root of the problem. None of this corruption and confusion and misrepresentation and suffering could happen without the DSM.

The DSM functions as the core of what John Sadler, professor of psychiatry and medical ethics, calls the Mental Health Medical Industrial Complex.[16] It's in the best interests of the stakeholders within that complex—drug companies, academic medical centers, the health care system, advertising and the media, and others—to protect the DSM. Psychiatrists, psychologists, researchers, and even the National Institutes of Health (NIH) still speak of DSM diagnoses as discrete disease entities.[17] Others defend the DSM by saying that although its diagnoses don't offer validity, they have "utility" meaning useful in a clinical setting.[18] Some uphold the DSM on the basis that its diagnoses can be understood as having "comparative validity" with "a correspondence to external reality."[19]

One of the largest stakeholders is biological psychiatry. Biopsychiatry may sound scientific, but it rests on theories, not findings. In over twenty years of research, it hasn't shown that DSM diagnoses are biological, yet the media, psychiatry, and pharma tell us they are.[20] Biopsychiatry rests on three claims: DSM diagnoses are heritable and/or genetic, caused by chemical imbalances, and visible on brain scans— none of which have been established. We don't know if DSM diagnoses really run in families or if they're caused by a flaw in one's genes.[21] Chemical imbalances are, at this point, little more than a cultural myth. And the effects of mental suffering can't be definitively observed on brain scans. Schizophrenia is the most oft-cited diagnosis used to try to prove the mental disorders are biological theory, but as many have pointed out, the studies referred to don't prove what they're said to prove.[22] In support of the schizophrenia-runs-in-families conclusion, studies rely on the results of earlier studies that had inconsistent results, some of which were influenced by the eugenics movement. Adoption studies often rely on researcher bias. If a researcher goes in believing a diagnosis is caused by biology, that researcher will draw biological results from the data; if a researcher favors the environmental explanation, that researcher will find the influence of environment *using the same data*. Despite the allure of the defective-gene theory, no single gene has been shown to cause any DSM diagnosis. (Psychiatry shrugs this off by saying, *Right, well, then it must be caused by multiple genes and it's just a matter of time until we obtain those findings*.) Brain-imaging may look convincing, but the enlargement of certain areas and the loss of gray matter in the brains of study participants can be caused by myriad factors. Even the APA admits neuroimaging can't be used in diagnosis.[23]

It's not enough to say—as many mental health professionals do—*Well, yes, the DSM is seriously flawed, even useless, but it's all we have*; the risks of labeling with an unfounded DSM diagnosis are too high. Stigma and self-stigma have so many adverse effects that it's hard to believe mental health professionals could justify using DSM diagnoses based on convenience (a.k.a. having supposed utility). Given how much damage DSM diagnoses can do, how can mental health professionals continue to use them without at the very least warning their patients and clients that the diagnoses they've received are hypothetical?

———

There are many types of lies: the white lie, little and supposedly harmless; the unspoken lie of omission; the cover-up; the bluff; the blue lie told in the name of the public good; exaggeration; confabulation, where a person lies because he doesn't know the truth; the lie said in jest; Plato's noble lie (also translated as the "magnificent myth"); the pathological lie; the polite lie; the half-truth. Saint Augustine distinguished between lies told out of pleasure versus those told out of harm.

Lying is common, maybe even "normal." (Ironically, pathological lying isn't a diagnosis found in the DSM though it is a symptom.) One study found that adults said they lie at least once a day.[24] Pinocchio had to lie to become a real boy. In Greek mythology, lying was considered a skill.

Which doesn't make it any less toxic. Christianity condemns it with its *Thou shalt not bear false witness*. In Buddhism, lying is a betrayal. Hannah Arendt said that lying destroys a society to the point that we can no longer believe in anything, which robs us of our ability to act.[25]

Were the therapist in New York and Dr. B and the psychiatrist in Iowa City and Dr. C and Dr. H and Dr. M lying when they handed me my diagnoses? Did they lie when they let me believe my diagnoses were caused by chemical imbalances? Should they have warned me that the biological theory supported by the NIH—which states "mental illness does indeed have a biological basis"—wasn't proven?[26]

Did they see their diagnoses as little white lies? Or did they view themselves as part of an elite guild enacting Plato's noble lie to advance their agenda? Did they tell themselves that covering up psychiatry's falsehoods would (certainly, probably, maybe) benefit the many? Or did they rationalize that their lies of omission were justified because they were merely allowing me to play a part in my treatment (code for *I should have known better*)? Did they tell themselves that since the brain-disease theory would (certainly, probably, maybe) be proven in the future, what was the harm in a little half-truth?

———

Right now, it falls to patients, mental health advocates, and potential patients (meaning everyone else) to create change. There's so much we can do.

We can make sure that those with DSM diagnoses know that those diagnoses are opinions, not facts. Even the authors of the DSM (quietly) confess they're unfounded. In a statement made by David Kupfer, chair of the DSM-5—a statement rarely, if ever mentioned in conversations about mental illness or by mental health organizations or in the media and certainly not by any of the doctors I saw—he admitted that DSM diagnoses aren't based on biological markers, are imprecise, and can't "be delivered with complete reliability and validity."[27] Mental illness exists, but what we call major depression, anxiety disorder, ADHD, etc., are creations of the DSM. They lead to the problem of false positives—overdiagnosis, misdiagnosis, and the mislabeling of normal distress as a mental disorder—a problem that's only getting worse.[28]

Influential public figures and professionals can take care with what they say and write. When celebrities speak out about their diagnoses, they can tell their fans that DSM diagnoses are, as yet, unproven. Journalists can explain (or, if we set the bar low, just mention) the complexities of saying that someone has any of the disorders listed in the DSM. Authors, editors, and publishers of books about mental health and mental-illness memoirs can do their research and qualify the terms they use.

We should talk about and tend to our mental and emotional health, but we can resist the urge to pathologize our thoughts and feelings and respect those in crisis. The phrase "everyone's a little mentally ill" doesn't destigmatize mental illness; it minimizes the conditions of those with serious mental illnesses, which can prevent resources going to them. This was the case with the Asperger's label. It was dropped from the DSM-5, in part, because, as task force chair of the DSM-5 David Kupfer said, some of the funding for autism research wasn't going toward those with severe autism.[29] We can reject "spectrums" that invite almost anyone to fall on them. The most recent edition of the DSM would like us to believe that mental illness is dimensional and that we're all just a doctor's office away from a diagnosis.

We can be more skeptical of psychiatrists. A recent Gallup poll reported that Americans' trust in psychiatrists' honesty and ethical standards *increased* between 2003 and 2019.[30] But given psychiatrists' lack of transparency about DSM diagnoses, have they really earned that trust? If a DSM diagnosis is unproven, invalid, possibly unreliable, and likely the result of lowered thresholds, what does that diagnosis really mean?

We can also question the role primary care physicians play in diagnosing mental illness. They shouldn't be allowed to do so without additional training and certification in mental health.

Knowing that DSM diagnoses haven't been proven to be chronic, we can consider suggested treatments more shrewdly. Physicians will need to explain how scientific studies on drug efficacy hold up without verifiable diagnoses. Psychiatric drug trials require all participants have the same diagnosis, e.g., depression, but if DSM diagnoses aren't valid, how can researchers know if participants have "depression"? Of what relevance are the results? If we accept a recommended treatment, we'll do so with the understanding that scientific studies having to do with the mind and behavior are often flawed and have been found to lack enduring value.[31]

We can demand not another DSM revision but full-on DSM reform. As former NIMH director Thomas Insel writes, "Patients with mental disorders deserve better."[32] We deserve DSM authors/task force members and leaders who don't take drug company money: 69 percent of the DSM-5's authors had financial ties to Big Pharma.[33]

Until psychiatry can provide real answers, we need to stop "spreading awareness" with false information about chemical imbalances and the other supposed causes of mental illness; instead, let's publicize the absence of validity and scientific evidence and the presence of lowered thresholds in the DSM, so people can make informed decisions about their diagnoses and treatment. (Psychiatry's defense might be along the lines of *Other fields of medicine have invalid diagnoses, too*. To that, we could answer, *Yes, but at least the majority of those are valid*.) If anyone can show that DSM diagnoses are scientifically proven, valid, and don't exhibit lowered thresholds, then by all means they should. In 2003, half a dozen members of MindFreedom International, a patient advocacy group that lobbied against forced treatment, went on a hunger strike and asked the APA, NAMI, and the US Office of the Surgeon General to provide any scientific evidence that proved, using a physical diagnostic exam, that any DSM diagnosis was a brain-based disease. No one could provide a single one. It's been nearly two decades, and we're still waiting.

———

Some organizations and mental health practitioners have been and are working toward reform. In 2011, the Society for Humanistic Psychology (SHP), a division of the APA, wrote an open letter to raise concerns about the ethical and scientific implications of the DSM-5. They were concerned about the lowering of diagnostic thresholds as well as the growing emphasis on biological theories: "In light of the growing empirical evidence that neurobiology does not fully account for the emergence of mental distress, as well as new longitudinal studies revealing long-term hazards of standard neurobiological (psychotropic) treatment, we believe that these changes [to the DSM] pose substantial risks." They were ignored. Since then, the SHP has argued for a paradigm shift that would admit to the DSM's pathologizing of "essentially 'normal' human responses" and has lobbied for the development of "scientifically sound and ethically principled" diagnostic manuals.[34]

The DSM-5 task force did invite the general public to weigh in on its revisions. Chair David Kupfer and Vice-Chair Darrel Regier created a webpage to take outside feedback into account, but it's unclear how or if that really happened.[35] The DSM-5 is now a digital, "living" document to which changes can be made at any time. Through an online portal, anyone can petition to have, say, obsessive compulsive disorder or autism removed. (Scientific data backing up suggested change is preferred but not necessary.) Although this democratizes the process by which feelings, thoughts, and behaviors are turned into illnesses and entered into the DSM, it doesn't exactly instill trust. Imagine the American Medical Association saying, *All diagnoses—cancer, diabetes, pneumonia, hypertension—could be gotten rid of, if you want. Or we could add a disorder, a disease, an illness based on your ideas and any data you can come up with. And if you think we should change the symptoms for a diagnosis or the level of dysfunction, just let us know because we've got precious little to go on.*

Individuals, organizations, and social media campaigns do try to warn people about DSM diagnoses. MindFreedom International has been trying to warn the public about the DSM since 1986. Robert Whitaker's Mad in America—which includes a podcast, a webzine, and educational courses—has been critiquing it since 2012. The *NO-DSM Diagnosis* campaign attempted a boycott of the DSM in 2013. More recently, Facebook groups and virtual conferences like "Drop the Disorder!" have called for us to challenge the DSM and improve how we refer to and speak about mental and emotional distress.

The critical psychiatry movement—not to be confused with antipsychiatry—has pointed to the lack of scientific evidence in psychiatric diagnoses and the skewed social and moral consequences of those diagnoses. Joanna Moncrieff, Sandra Steingard, and others attempt to cull the best of psychiatry while acknowledging its worst.[36]

What's the alternative to the DSM? Other diagnostic systems aren't yet viable. The WHO's *International Classification of Diseases* doesn't suffer from the same financial conflicts as the DSM does and has fewer diagnoses, but it leaves even more to the discretion of the clinician and is thought to be less accurate. The NIMH's Research Domain Criteria (RDoC) focuses on degrees of dysfunction, which could lead to more diagnostic precision; currently, however, the RDoC is still a research framework, not a diagnostic guide intended for clinical practice.[37]

Suggestions, made by Nassir Ghaemi, an attending psychiatrist and professor of psychiatry and pharmacology at Tufts University School of Medicine, and others advocate for reducing the number of DSM diagnoses. Ghaemi has said we should return to the diagnoses from the Feigner criteria, remove the rest, and keep only those diagnoses that have the most viable research.[38] No more inventing of diagnoses and clustering of symptoms and pathologizing emotions, thoughts, and behaviors based on the opinions and ideas of APA members and other mental health professionals.

There are no easy answers, but we need to start having the right conversation, one that focuses on the dangers of the DSM.

———

Even if we find an alternative to the DSM, it won't be easy to counteract the damage done by the DSM. Too many psychiatrists won't admit the truth. One need only read *Shrinks: The Untold Story of Psychiatry* by Jeffrey Lieberman, former head of the APA.

Lieberman glosses over the fact that no DSM diagnosis is scientifically valid and proclaims that psychiatry is a medical specialty on the verge of greatness: "[P]sychiatry is finally taking its rightful place in the medical community after a long sojourn in the scientific wilderness."[39] He boasts that during the DSM-5 revisions, the task force "adopted the strictest ethics policy" and that psychiatrists' dealings with drug companies "must be transparent, rigorously monitored, and without conflicts of interest."[40] His solution wasn't that anyone stop taking drug company money and inventing diagnoses, just admit they took the money—at least most of the time.[41] Lieberman's own close ties to Big Pharma (fifteen companies, according to infectious disease specialist and writer Judith Stone) and inaccurate findings about the effectiveness of antipsychotics seem to trouble him not at all.[42]

Like many psychiatrists, Lieberman could be said to suffer from hubris. Biederman certainly did. During his 2009 deposition, Biederman was asked about his rank at Harvard Medical School. He answered, "Full professor." When asked what was above that, Biederman said, "God."[43]

Dr. M exuded hubris—albeit subtly. His excessive self-confidence revealed itself in his need to be right about my diagnosis. If asked, he, like many psychologists and psychiatrists, might have claimed that it had nothing to do with the DSM because the DSM doesn't reflect how he actually conducts his practice. But instead of helping me understand that my diagnosis (*my* diagnosis) was hypothetical, he made it more real. He failed to heed the advice found in *The Intelligent Clinician's Guide to the DSM-5*: "In the absence of independent measures ... we cannot be sure that *any* category in the manual is valid. We should not therefore think of current psychiatric diagnoses as 'real' in the same way as medical diseases. Also, listing [diagnoses] in a manual does not make them real ... [P]sychiatrists must make diagnoses, but they do not need to reify them. They are best advised to stay humble and to avoid hubris."[44]

I wouldn't have minded any of my diagnoses if he and Dr. H and Dr. C and Dr. B and the psychiatrists in Iowa City had been honest—if just one, aside from Dr. R, had admitted to not knowing: *It could be major depression (or an anxiety disorder [or ADHD (or bipolar or ...)]), but those diagnoses have never been proven. It's a theoretical diagnosis, an idea about a diagnosis, you can choose to accept or not. Oh, and here are drugs you can take, which are equally unproven. Oh, and you may have terrible side effects and you may never be able to go off this one drug and* . . . I may still have accepted the diagnoses I received. Given the severity of what I was experiencing, I might have taken the medications prescribed. But my decisions wouldn't have been based on lies of omission.

———

I sit at one of the tables in my creative writing workshop. The discussion is animated. The class is made up of juniors and seniors who don't have much confidence in their writing but are very, very sociable. They've bonded over the quarter and come to trust each other.

The story we're workshopping is by a student whose talent astounds me. He seems to have an internal understanding of characterization and description. His punctuation and grammar skills are excellent.

The main character in the story is an antihero—rough and un-pleasant. By the end, he becomes violent. His violence is explained not as a complicated mix of factors, impulses, desires, socioeconomic conditions, skewed beliefs, and mistakes but with two words: mental illness.

I sip my water and listen as the students tell the writer what they think is working in the story. After they share their thoughts for revi-sion, I ask them if the character has to have a mental illness. They look at me like I've asked them to stop scrolling on their phones forever: total incomprehension.

One student says, "It explains him and what he does."

I ask if that's true. Do they understand the character better with that identity?

Some say no; others stick with yes.

After class, I walk through the hallway crowded with students. Three young men in front of me jostle each other. Someone shouts. A young woman passes with tears in her eyes.

All I have is the knowledge that DSM diagnoses are easy to get and aren't to be trusted. More than 46 percent of American adults and 20 percent of children and adolescents will receive a DSM diagnosis in their lifetimes.[45] Picture a stadium full of adults. Half of them will think they have a mental illness. Imagine a playground full of children. One in five of them will be told they are mentally ill.

Few, if any, of them will be told that their diagnoses come from a book that's primarily a collection of relatively common behaviors, thoughts, and emotions that have been ordered and reordered and pathologized. Or that those diagnoses can't be proven to exist and are opinions, not facts. (As mentioned, exceptions include dementia and rare chromosomal disorders.)

Because that would make people wary, and the DSM is designed to diagnose as many people as possible.[46] It does this by adding new diagnoses and subtypes (e.g., binge-eating disorder) and including milder versions of diagnoses (e.g., bipolar II) and lowering standards to include and keep the most unreliable of diagnoses (e.g., generalized anxiety disorder and major depressive disorder).[47] And by replacing words. And inserting punctuation—say, a slash.

I give you this: Before you accept a DSM diagnosis, pause. That doesn't mean you don't seek treatment or take medication or ultimately decide that having a diagnosis, no matter how tenuous (at least for now), serves you, but you do so knowing the truth.

Acknowledgments

It's beyond rare to find an agent who sees the potential in a book and backs it 100 percent, and even rarer to get an editor who can zero in on what a book needs. I was lucky enough to have both. Thank you to my agent, Kim Witherspoon, and to my editor, Sydney Rogers. Thank you also to Maria Whelan and everyone at InkWell Management and Gideon Weil and everyone at HarperOne. To Andrea Robinson, Shelby Brewster, and Kerri Marikakis for editorial guidance. To Ray Emerick for listening to the first draft of this book, which I haphazardly recorded. To Mary Hickman for listening to me during the writing of this and beyond. To Sydney Rhinehart and Chloe Korn for your comments and research assistance. To Noah Isackson and Michele Morano for your feedback and encouragement. To Alice Markham-Cantor, the best fact-checker in the world. Very special thanks to Cheri Lucas Rowlands and *Longreads*, Marisa Siegel and *The Rumpus*, and Hannah Webster and *Michigan Quarterly Review* for believing in and publishing early versions of parts of this work.

Finally, to my family, who supported me and never asked for any of this, and to Greg Baker (1947–2000), who first taught me the beauty of a punctuated life.

Notes

Prologue

1. Philip Horsfield *et al.*, "Self-Labeling as Having a Mental or Physical Illness: The Effects of Stigma and Implications for Help-Seeking," *Social Psychiatry and Psychiatric Epidemiology* 55 (2020): 907–16, https://doi.org/10.1007/s00127-019-01787-7.

2. Allan V. Horwitz, *DSM: A History of Psychiatry's Bible* (Baltimore, MD: Johns Hopkins University Press, 2021), 5.

3. S. Nassir Ghaemi, "Why DSM-III, IV, and 5 Are Unscientific," *Psychiatric Times*, October 14, 2013, https://www.psychiatrictimes.com/view/why-dsm-iii-iv-and-5-are-unscientific; James Davies, "How Voting and Consensus Created the Diagnostic and Statistical Manual of Mental Disorders (DSM-III)," *Anthropology & Medicine* 24, no. 1 (2017): 32–46, https://doi.org/10.1080/13648470.2016.1226684.

4. Gary Greenberg, "The Rats of N.I.M.H.," *The New Yorker*, May 16, 2013, https://www.newyorker.com/tech/annals-of-technology/the-rats-of-n-i-m-h; Stijn Vanheule, *Diagnosis and the DSM: A Critical Review* (Basingstoke: Palgrave Macmillan, 2014).

5. Insel quoted in Andrew Scull, "Mad Science: The Treatment of Mental Illness Fails to Progress [Excerpt]," *Scientific American*, April 16, 2015, https://www.scientificamerican.com/article/mad-science-the-treatment-of-mental-illness-fails-to-progress-excerpt/.

6. Awais Aftab, "Conversations in Critical Psychiatry: Allen Frances, MD," *Psychiatric Times* 36, no. 10 (May 22, 2019), https://www.psychiatrictimes.com/view/conversations-critical-psychiatry-allen-frances-md.

7. Steven E. Hyman, "Revitalizing Psychiatric Therapeutics," *Neuropsychopharmacology* 39 (2014): 220–29, https://www.nature.com/articles/npp2013181.

8. Joel Paris, "Diagnostic Validity," chap. 5 in *The Intelligent Clinician's Guide to the DSM-5*, 2nd ed. (New York: Oxford University Press, 2015); Thomas Insel, "Transforming Diagnosis," NIMH Director's Blog, April 29, 2013, http://psychrights.org/2013/130429NIMHTransformingDiagnosis.htm.

9. Ahmed Aboraya, "The Reliability of Psychiatric Diagnoses," *Psychiatry* 4, no. 1 (January 2007): 22–25; S. Nassir Ghaemi, "Requiem for DSM," *Psychiatric Times* 30, no. 7 (July 17, 2013), https://www.psychiatrictimes.com/view/requiem-dsm.

10. Determining the number of diagnoses in the DSM depends on how many subtypes you count and if you include Not Otherwise Specified (NOS), which should be counted because it's often used to diagnose those who don't fit the diagnosis but get one anyway.

The calculations used here are from Roger K. Blashfield, et al., "The Cycle of Classification: DSM-I through DSM-5," *Annual Review of Clinical Psychology* 10 (2014): 25–51, https://doi.org/10.1146/annurev-clinpsy-032813-153639.

11. Ghaemi, "Requiem for DSM." Hannah S. Decker, "Corporate Profits and the DSMs: The Case of the Tobacco Industry," *Psychiatric Times*, May 23, 2013, https://www.psych iatrictimes.com/view/corporate-profits-and-dsms-case-tobacco-industry; Brendan I. Koerner, "First, You Market the Disease . . . Then You Push the Pills to Treat It," *The Guardian*, July 30, 2002, https://www.theguardian.com/news/2002/jul/30/medicineand health.

12. Council for Evidence-Based Psychiatry, "Diagnostic System Lacks Validity," revised March 15, 2014, http://cepuk.org/unrecognised-facts/diagnostic-system-lacks-validity/.

13. Ghaemi, "Requiem for DSM."

14. Keith Houston, "The Rise and Fall of the Pilcrow, Part 1," *Slate*, September 25, 2013, https://slate.com/human-interest/2013/09/the-pilcrow-how-the-paragraph -punctuation-mark-evolved-from-ancient-greece-and-rome.html; Keith Houston, "The Mysterious Origins of Punctuation," BBC Culture, September 2, 2015, https://www .bbc.com/culture/article/20150902-the-mysterious-origins-of-punctuation.

1. The Weight of a Comma

1. Karen Blazer, "Seventeen Magazine Covers," Pinterest, *Seventeen*, March 1975, accessed June 2020, https://www.pinterest.com/pin/8233211793271948/; Lori A. Smolin and Mary B. Grosvenor, *Nutrition and Eating Disorders* (Philadelphia: Chelsea House Publishers, 2009).

2. Carol Lawson, "Anorexia: It's Not a New Disease," *New York Times*, December 8, 1985, https://www.nytimes.com/1985/12/08/style/anorexia-it-s-not-a-new-disease.html; A. R. Lucas *et al.*, "50-Year Trends in the Incidence of Anorexia Nervosa in Rochester, Minn.: A Population-Based Study," *American Journal of Psychiatry* 148, no. 7 (July 1991): 917–22, https://doi.org/10.1176/ajp.148.7.917.

3. Bridget Dolan, "Cross-Cultural Aspects of Anorexia Nervosa and Bulimia: A Review," *International Journal of Eating Disorders* 10, no. 1 (January 1991): 67–79, https:// doi.org/10.1002/1098-108X(199101)10:1<67::AID-EAT2260100108>3.0.CO;2-N.

4. Walter Vandereycken and Ron Van Deth, "Who Was the First to Describe Anorexia Nervosa: Gull or Lasègue?," *Psychological Medicine* 19, no. 4 (1989): 837–45, https:// doi.org/10.1017/s0033291700005559.

5. Anthony Storr, *Freud: A Very Short Introduction* (Oxford: Oxford University Press, 2001), 118; Liliana Dell'Osso *et al.*, "Historical Evolution of the Concept of Anorexia Nervosa and Relationships with Orthorexia Nervosa, Autism, and Obsessive-Compulsive Spectrum," *Neuropsychiatric Disease and Treatment* 12 (2016): 1651–60, https://doi.org/10.2147/NDT.S108912; C. Mushatt, "Anorexia Nervosa: A Psychoanalytic Commentary," *International Journal of Psychoanalytic Psychotherapy* 9 (1982): 257–65.

6. Sharon Johnson, "Relationships: Anorexia as Family Problem," *New York Times*, April 1987.

7. Jana Evans Braziel and Kathleen LeBesco, *Bodies Out of Bounds: Fatness and Transgression* (Berkeley: University of California Press, 2001).

8. Peg Byron, "Heat and Anorexia Your Health: Summer Means Heat Is on for Anorexics," United Press International, May 21, 1988, https://www.upi.com/Archives /1988/05/21/Heat-and-anorexia-Your-Health-Summer-means-heat-is-on-for-anorexics /9802580190400/.

9. Dina L. Borzekowski *et al.*, "e-Ana and e-Mia: A Content Analysis of Pro–Eating Disorder Web Sites," *American Journal of Public Health* 100, no. 8 (August 2010): 1526–34, https://doi.org/10.2105/AJPH.2009.172700.

10. Randy L. Schmidt, *Yesterday Once More*, 2nd ed. (Chicago: Chicago Review Press, 2012).

11. D. L. Franko *et al.*, "What Predicts Suicide Attempts in Women with Eating Disorders?," *Psychological Medicine* 34, no. 5 (July 2004): 843–53, https://doi.org/10.1017/s0033291703001545.

12. Hilde Bruch, "Perceptual and Conceptual Disturbances in Anorexia Nervosa," *Psychosomatic Medicine* 24, no. 2 (March 1962): 187–94, https://doi.org/10.1097/00006842-196203000-00009.

13. Ellen Watkins and Lucy Serpell, "The Psychological Effects of Short-Term Fasting in Healthy Women," *Frontiers in Nutrition* 3 (2016): 27, https://doi.org/10.3389%2Ffnut.2016.00027.

14. Amarish Davé, "Could Skipping Breakfast Relieve Depression?," PsychCentral, October 30, 2016, https://psychcentral.com/lib/could-skipping-breakfast-relieve-depression/; Yifan Zhang *et al.*, "The Effects of Calorie Restriction in Depression and Potential Mechanisms," *Current Neuropharmacology* 13, no. 4 (2015): 536–42, https://doi.org/10.2174/1570159x13666150326003852.

15. John Smyth, *A Paterne of True Prayer*, 1605.

16. New York University, "Professor Replicates Famous Marshmallow Test, Makes New Observations," ScienceDaily, May 25, 2018, www.sciencedaily.com/releases/2018/05/180525095226.htm.

17. Dell'Osso *et al.*, "Historical Evolution of the Concept of Anorexia Nervosa."

18. Aboraya, "The Reliability of Psychiatric Diagnoses."

2. Consider the Colon

1. Mike Slade and Eleanor Longden, "Empirical Evidence about Recovery and Mental Health," *BMC Psychiatry* 15 (2015): article 285, https://doi.org/10.1186/s12888-015-0678-4.

2. National Alliance on Mental Illness, "Can People Recover from Mental Illness? Is There a Cure?," National Alliance on Mental Illness, https://www.nami.org/FAQ/General-Information-FAQ/Can-people-recover-from-mental-illness-Is-there-a.

3. Allan V. Horwitz, "Creating an Age of Depression: The Social Construction and Consequences of the Major Depression Diagnosis," *Society and Mental Health* 1, no. 1 (March 2011): 41–54, https://doi.org/10.1177/2156869310393986; Allan V. Horwitz, "How an Age of Anxiety Became an Age of Depression," *The Milbank Quarterly* 88, no. 1 (2010): 112–38, https://doi.org/10.1111/j.1468-0009.2010.00591.x/.

4. Ken Kusmer, "Prozac, the Blockbuster Antidepressant Drug," *AP News*, February 12, 1997, https://apnews.com/7e8db70ea62ae0cb44c22f3deb1bb5a0.

5. Alix Spiegel, "The Dictionary of Disorder," *The New Yorker* 80, no. 41 (2005): 56–63.

6. Owen Whooley, *On the Heels of Ignorance: Psychiatry and the Politics of Not Knowing* (Chicago: University of Chicago Press, 2019).

7. Bassam Khoury, Ellen J. Langer, and Francesco Pagnini, "The DSM: Mindful Science or Mindless Power? A Critical Review," *Frontiers in Psychology* 5, no. 602 (June 17, 2014), https://doi.org/10.3389/fpsyg.2014.00602; Kenneth S. Kendler, Rodrigo A. Muñoz, and George Murphy, "The Development of the Feighner Criteria: A Historical Perspective," *The American Journal of Psychiatry* 167, no. 2 (February 2010): 134–42, https://doi.org/10.1176/appi.ajp.2009.09081155.

8. Diogo Telles-Correia, Sérgio Saraiva, and Jorge Gonçalves, "Mental Disorder—The Need for an Accurate Definition," *Frontiers in Psychiatry* 9, no. 64 (March 12, 2018), https://doi.org/10.3389/fpsyt.2018.00064.

9. Edward Shorter, "The History of DSM," in *Making the DSM-5: Concepts and Controversies*, ed. Joel Paris and James Phillips (New York: Springer Nature, 2013), 3–19, https://doi.org/10.1007/978-1-4614-6504-1.

10. Nancy C. Andreasen, *The Broken Brain: The Biological Revolution in Psychiatry* (New York: HarperPerennial, 1984), 29–30.

11. Kirsten Weir, "The Roots of Mental Illness," *Monitor on Psychology* 43, no. 6 (June 2012): 30, https://www.apa.org/monitor/2012/06/roots; National Institutes of Health, "Information about Mental Illness and the Brain," *NIH Curriculum Supplement Series* (Bethseda, MD: Bethesda (MD): National Institutes of Health, 2007), https://www.ncbi.nlm.nih.gov/books/NBK20369/.

12. Mark L. Ruffalo, "Psychiatric Diagnosis 2.0: The Myth of the Symptom Checklist," *Psychology Today*, June 14, 2020, https://www.psychologytoday.com/us/blog/freud-fluoxetine/202006/psychiatric-diagnosis-20-the-myth-the-symptom-checklist.

13. T. Patil and J Giordano, "On the ontological assumptions of the medical model of psychiatry: philosophical considerations and pragmatic tasks," *Philos Ethics Humanit Med* 5, no. 3 (2010). https://doi.org/10.1186/1747-5341-5-3.

14. Paul Hoff, "On Reification of Mental Illness: Historical and Conceptual Issues from Emil Kraepelin and Eugen Bleuler to DSM-5," chap. 14 in *Philosophical Issues in Psychiatry IV: Classification of Psychiatric Illness*, ed. Kenneth S. Kendler and Josef Parnas (Oxford: Oxford University Press, 2017), https://doi.org/10.1093/med/9780198796022.003.0014.

15. Gary Greenberg, *The Book of Woe: The DSM and the Unmaking of Psychiatry* (New York: Blue Rider Press, 2013), 37, Kindle.

16. Allen Frances, *Saving Normal: An Insider's Revolt against Out-of-Control Psychiatric Diagnosis, DSM-5, Big Pharma, and the Medicalization of Ordinary Life* (New York: William Morrow, 2013), 63, Kindle.

17. Gerald N. Grob, "Presidential Address: Psychiatry's Holy Grail: The Search for the Mechanisms of Mental Diseases," *Bulletin of the History of Medicine* 72, no. 2 (Summer 1998): 211.

18. American Psychiatric Association, *Diagnostic and Statistical Manual of Mental Disorders* (Arlington, VA: American Psychiatric Association, 1952).

19. Shorter, "The History of DSM."

20. Shadia Kawa and James Giordano, "A Brief Historicity of the *Diagnostic and Statistical Manual of Mental Disorders*: Issues and Implications for the Future of Psychiatric Canon and Practice," *Philosophy, Ethics, and Humanities in Medicine* 7, no. 2 (January 2012): article 2, https://doi.org/10.1186/1747-5341-7-2.

21. Paul T. Wilson and Robert L. Spitzer, "Major Changes in Psychiatric Nomenclature: Reconciling Existing Psychiatric Medical Records with the New American Psychiatric Association Diagnostic and Statistical Manual of Mental Disorders," *Psychiatric Services* 19, no. 6 (June 1968): 169–74.

22. Rick Mayes and Allan V. Horwitz, "DSM-III and the Revolution in the Classification of Mental Illness," *Journal of the History of the Behavioral Sciences* 41, no. 3 (2005): 249–67; Telles-Correia, Saraiva, and Gonçalves, "Mental Disorder"; Hema Venigalla *et al.*, "An Update on Biomarkers in Psychiatric Disorders—Are We Aware, Do We Use in Our Clinical Practice?," *Mental Health in Family Medicine* 13, (2017): 471–79,

http://www.mhfmjournal.com/pdf/an-update-on-biomarkers-in-psychiatric-disorders--are-we-aware-do-we-use-in-our-clinical-practice.pdf.

23. Horwitz, *DSM*, 49, 52.
24. Joel Paris, "The Ideology Behind DSM-5," in *Making the DSM-5: Concepts and Controversies* (New York: Springer Nature, 2013), https://doi-org.turing.library.northwestern.edu/10.1007/978-1-4614-6504-1_3.
25. Jerome C. Wakefield, "The Concept of Mental Disorder: Diagnostic Implications of the Harmful Dysfunction Analysis," *World Psychiatry: Official Journal of the World Psychiatric Association (WPA)* 6, no. 3 (2007): 149–56.
26. Gary Greenberg, "Inside the Battle to Define Mental Illness," *Wired*, December 27, 2010, https://www.wired.com/2010/12/ff-dsmv/.
27. María A. Oquendo *et al.*, "Issues for DSM-V: Suicidal Behavior as a Separate Diagnosis on a Separate Axis," *The American Journal of Psychiatry* 165, no. 11 (November 2008): 1383–84, https://doi.org/10.1176/appi.ajp.2008.08020281.
28. Oquendo *et al.*, "Issues for DSM-V."
29. Mary Frances Kennedy Fisher, *The Art of Eating: 50th Anniversary Edition* (Boston: Mariner Books, 2004), 490, Kindle.
30. William Styron, *Darkness Visible: A Memoir of Madness* (New York: Open Road Integrated Media, 2010), 14, Kindle.
31. Styron, *Darkness Visible*, 22.
32. Styron, *Darkness Visible*, 33.
33. Styron, *Darkness Visible*, 35.
34. Christopher Mulvey, "The English Project's History of English Punctuation," The English Project, http://www.englishproject.org/resources/english-project's-history-english-punctuation.

3. Suspension Points

1. Alison Flood, "Unfinished Story . . . How the Ellipsis Arrived in English Literature," *The Guardian*, October 20, 2015, https://www.theguardian.com/books/2015/oct/20/unfinished-story-how-the-ellipsis-arrived-in-english-literature.
2. Anne Toner, *Ellipses in English Literature* (New York: Cambridge University Press, 2015), 7, Kindle.
3. Boris Tabakoff and Paula L. Hoffman, "The Neurobiology of Alcohol Consumption and Alcoholism: An Integrative History," *Pharmacology Biochemistry and Behavior* 113 (November 2013): 20–37, https://doi.org/10.1016/j.pbb.2013.10.009.
4. Thomas F. Babor, "The Classification of Alcoholics: Typology Theories from the 19th Century to the Present," *Alcohol Health and Research World* 20, no. 1 (1996): 6–14, https://www.ncbi.nlm.nih.gov/pmc/articles/PMC6876530/.
5. J. Douglas Sellman *et al.*, "DSM-5 Alcoholism: A 60-Year Perspective," *Australian and New Zealand Journal of Psychiatry* 48, no. 6 (2014): 507–11, https://doi.org/10.1177/0004867414532849.
6. Sean M. Robinson and Bryon Adinoff, "The Classification of Substance Use Disorders: Historical, Contextual, and Conceptual Considerations," *Behavioral Sciences* 6, no. 3 (2016): 18, https://doi.org/10.3390/bs6030018.
7. Francesco Bartoli *et al.*, "From DSM-IV to DSM-5 Alcohol Use Disorder: An Overview of Epidemiological Data," *Addictive Behaviors* 41 (February 2015): 46–50, https://doi.org/10.1016/j.addbeh.2014.09.029.

8. Center for Substance Abuse Treatment, *Managing Chronic Pain in Adults with or in Recovery from Substance Use Disorders*, Treatment Improvement Protocol Series 54, exhibit 2–6, *DSM-IV-TR Criteria for Substance Abuse and Substance Dependence*, (Rockville, MD: Substance Abuse and Mental Health Services Administration, 2012), https://www.ncbi.nlm.nih.gov/books/NBK92053/table/ch2.t5/.

9. Susan Baur, "A Disease So Grievous, So Common," chap. 2 in *Hypochondria: Woeful Imaginings* (Berkeley: University of California Press, 1989).

10. Stephen Heath, "Hypochondria: Medical Condition, Creative Malady," *Brain* 134, no. 4 (April 2011): 1244–49, https://doi.org/10.1093/brain/awr006.

11. John Mullan, "Hypochondria and Hysteria: Sensibility and the Physicians," *The Eighteenth Century* 25, no. 2 (1984): 141–74, http://www.jstor.org/stable/41467321.

12. Justine Nienke Pannekoek and Dan J. Stein, "Diagnosis and Classification of Hypochondriasis," in *Hypochondriasis and Health Anxiety: A Guide for Clinicians*, ed. Vladan Starcevic and Russell Noyes (Oxford: Oxford University Press, 2014), 28–38, https://doi.org/10.1093/med/9780199996865.003.0003.

13. Baur, "A Disease So Grievous, So Common"; Arthur J. Barsky *et al.*, "A Prospective 4- to 5-Year Study of DSM-III-R Hypochondriasis," *Archives of General Psychiatry* 55, no. 8 (1998): 737–44, https://doi.org/10.1001/archpsyc.55.8.737.

14. Francis Creed, "New Research on Medically Unexplained Symptoms—Much Remains to Be Done Before *DSM V* and *ICD-10* Can Provide a Satisfactory New Classification," *Journal of Psychosomatic Research* 66, no. 5 (May 2009): 359–61, https://doi.org/10.1016/j.jpsychores.2009.02.005; Juan Francisco Rodríguez-Testal, Cristina Senín-Calderón, and Salvador Perona-Garcelán, "From DSM-IV-TR to DSM-5: Analysis of Some Changes," *International Journal of Clinical and Health Psychology* 14, no. 3 (2014): 221–31, https://doi.org/10.1016/j.ijchp.2014.05.002.

15. B. A. Fallon *et al.*, "Hypochondriasis and Its Relationship to Obsessive-Compulsive Disorder," *Psychiatric Clinics of North America* 23, no. 3 (September 2000): 605–16, https://doi.org/10.1016/s0193-953x(05)70183-0; Bunmi O. Olatunji, Brett J. Deacon, and Jonathan S. Abramowitz, "Is Hypochondriasis an Anxiety Disorder?," *British Journal of Psychiatry* 194, no. 6 (June 2009): 481–82, https://doi.org/10.1192/bjp.bp.108.061085.

16. David Batho, "Addiction as Powerlessness? Choice, Compulsion, and 12-Step Programmes," (EOP green paper, The Ethics of Powerlessness, University of Essex, November 7, 2017), https://powerlessness.essex.ac.uk/addictionaspowerlessness_green_paper; Buddy T. "Recognizing Alcoholism as a Disease," Verywell Mind, March 17, 2021, https://www.verywellmind.com/alcoholism-as-a-disease-63292; Gabrielle Glaser, "The Irrationality of Alcoholics Anonymous," *The Atlantic*, April 2015, https://www.theatlantic.com/magazine/archive/2015/04/the-irrationality-of-alcoholics-anonymous/386255/; Marlene Oscar-Berman and Ksenija Marinkovic, "Alcoholism and the Brain: An Overview," *Alcohol Research and Health* 27, no. 2 (2003): 125–33, https://pubs.niaaa.nih.gov/publications/arh27-2/125-133.htm; Melissa Carmona, ed., "Why Is Alcoholism Considered a Chronic Disease?," The Recovery Village, updated January 25, 2021, https://www.therecoveryvillage.com/alcohol-abuse/faq/alcoholism-considered-chronic-disease/; "Is Alcoholism a Disease?," Recovery Centers of America, https://recoverycentersofamerica.com/alcohol-abuse-addiction/is-alcoholism-a-disease/; Ernest Kurtz, "Alcoholics Anonymous and the Disease Concept of Alcoholism," *Alcoholism Treatment Quarterly* 20, no. 3–4 (2002): 5–39, https://doi.org/10.1300/J020v20n03_02; "AA as a Resource for the Health Care Professional," Alcoholics Anonymous, https://www.aa.org/pages/en_US/aa-as-a-resource-for-the-health-car-professional; Bill Wilson, "Talk to the National Clergy Conference on

Alcoholism," http://westbalto.a-1associates.com/LETS_ASK_BILL/wilsonstalktothe clergy.htm.

17. George E. Vaillant and Susanne Hiller-Sturmhöfel, "The Natural History of Alcoholism," *Alcohol Health and Research World* 20, no. 3 (1996): 152–61, https://www.ncbi.nlm.nih .gov/pmc/articles/PMC6876506/.

18. Anne Harrington, "Beyond Phrenology: Localization Theory in the Modern Era," in *The Enchanted Loom: Chapters in the History of Neuroscience*, ed. Pietro Corsi (New York: Oxford University Press, 1991), 207–39.

19. Storr, *Freud: A Very Short Introduction*.

20. G. N. Grob, "Origins of DSM-I: A Study in Appearance and Reality," *American Journal of Psychiatry* 148, no. 4 (April 1991): 421–31, https://doi.org/10.1176/ajp.148.4.421.

21. Horwitz, *DSM*, 20.

22. Ruth Leys, "Types of One: Adolf Meyer's Life Chart and the Representation of Individuality," *Representations* 34 (April 1991): 1–28, https://doi.org/10.2307/2928768.

23. Arthur C. Houts, "Fifty Years of Psychiatric Nomenclature: Reflections on the 1943 War Department Technical Bulletin, Medical 203," *Journal of Clinical Psychology* 56, no. 7 (July 2000): 935–67, https://doi.org/10.1002/1097-4679(200007)56:7<935::AID -JCLP11>3.0.CO;2-8.

24. *Newsweek* Staff, "Remembering the Great American Writer Ernest Hemingway on His Birthday," *Newsweek*, July 21, 2015, https://www.newsweek.com/ernest-heming ways-birthday-july-21-2015-355999; Nathan Heller, "Hemingway," Slate, March 16, 2012, https://slate.com/culture/2012/03/ernest-hemingway-how-the-great-american -novelist-became-the-literary-equivalent-of-the-nike-swoosh.html.

25. Toni Morrison, "The Color Fetish," *The New Yorker*, September 14, 2017, https://www .newyorker.com/books/page-turner/the-color-fetish.

26. Matthew Feldman, "Make It Crude: Ezra Pound's Antisemitic Propaganda for the BUF and PNF," *Holocaust Studies* 15, no. 1–2 (2009): 59–77, https://doi.org/10.1080/17 504902.2009.11087226.

27. Linda Thraysbule, "Alcohol Releases the Brain's 'Feel Good' Chemicals," LiveScience, May 30, 2013, https://www.livescience.com/36084-alcohol-releases-endorphins -brain.html.

28. American Addiction Centers, "How Are Emotional Effects of Alcohol Explained?" Alcohol.org, accessed July 1, 2020, https://www.alcohol.org/guides/alcohol-fueled -emotions/.

29. Ivan Rusyn and Ramon Bataller, "Alcohol and Toxicity," *Journal of Hepatology* 59, no. 2 (August 2013): 387–88, https://doi.org/10.1016/j.jhep.2013.01.035.

30. Nicholas W. Gilpin and George F. Koob, "Neurobiology of Alcohol Dependence: Focus on Motivational Mechanisms," National Institute on Alcohol Abuse and Alcoholism, https://pubs.niaaa.nih.gov/publications/arh313/185-195.htm.

31. Northpoint Staff, "9 Signs of Alcohol Poisoning," Northpoint Recovery, September 27, 2017, https://www.northpointrecovery.com/blog/9-signs-alcohol-poisoning/.

32. Mayo Clinic Staff, "Illness Anxiety Disorder," Mayo Clinic, April 19, 2021, https:// www.mayoclinic.org/diseases-conditions/illness-anxiety-disorder/symptoms-causes /syc-20373782.

33. UNC Health Talk, "Heavy Drinking Rewires Brain, Increasing Susceptibility to Anxiety Problems," UNC Health, September 4, 2012, https://healthtalk.unchealthcare.org /heavy-drinking-rewires-brain-increasing-susceptibility-to-anxiety-problems/.

4. Un-joined

1. Elizabeth von Muggenthaler, "The Felid Purr: A Healing Mechanism?," *The Journal of the Acoustical Society of America* 110, no. 2666 (2001), https://doi.org/10.1121/1.4777098.

2. Michael Shermer, "Five Fallacies of Grief: Debunking Psychological Stages," *Scientific American*, November 1, 2008, https://www.scientificamerican.com/article/five-fallacies-of-grief/.

3. "Grief Cat," Google Search Engine, 43.9 million results, July 2020, https://www.google.com/search?q=grief+cat.

4. Karl Sudi *et al.*, "Anorexia Athletica," *Nutrition* 20, no. 7–8 (July–August 2004): 657–61, https://doi.org/10.1016/j.nut.2004.04.019.

5. Caroline Meyer *et al.*, "The Compulsive Exercise Test: Confirmatory Factor Analysis and Links with Eating Psychopathology among Women with Clinical Eating Disorders," *Journal of Eating Disorders* 4, (2016): article 22, https://doi.org/10.1186/s40337-016-0113-3.

6. Horwitz, "How an Age of Anxiety"; Democritus Junior, *The Anatomy of Melancholy* (Project Gutenberg, 2004), https://www.gutenberg.org/files/10800/10800-h/10800-h.htm; G. E. Berrios, "Melancholia and Depression during the 19th Century: A Conceptual History," *British Journal of Psychiatry* 153, no. 3 (1988): 298–304, https://doi.org/10.1192/bjp.153.3.298.

7. Allan V. Horwitz and Jerome C. Wakefield, *The Loss of Sadness: How Psychiatry Transformed Normal Sorrow into Depressive Disorder* (Cary: Oxford University Press, 2007).

8. Anne Harrington, *Mind Fixers: Psychiatry's Troubled Search for the Biology of Mental Illness* (New York: W. W. Norton and Company, 2019), 202, 204–6, 244, Kindle.

9. Harrington, *Mind Fixers*.

10. Horwitz and Wakefield, *Loss of Sadness*.

11. Frances, *Saving Normal*, 154.

12. Paula J. Clayton, James A. Halikas, and William L. Maurice, "The Depression of Widowhood," *British Journal of Psychiatry* 120, no. 554 (1972): 71–77, https://doi.org/10.1192/bjp.120.554.71.

13. Horwitz and Wakefield, *Loss of Sadness*, 213.

14. American Psychiatric Association, *Diagnostic and Statistical Manual of Mental Disorders*, 4th ed. (*DSM-IV*) (Washington, DC: American Psychiatric Association, 1994), 91.

15. Frances, *Saving Normal*.

5. Ask Your Doctor

1. Hal Arkowitz and Scott O. Lilienfeld, "Is There Really an Autism Epidemic?," *Scientific American*, August 1, 2012, https://www.scientificamerican.com/article/is-there-really-an-autism-epidemic/.

2. Morton Ann Gernsbacher, Michelle Dawson, and H. Hill Goldsmith, "Three Reasons Not to Believe in an Autism Epidemic," *Current Directions in Psychological Science* 14, no. 2 (April 2005): 55–58, https://doi.org/10.1111/j.0963-7214.2005.00334.x; Centers for Disease Control and Prevention, "Autism Spectrum Disorder Data and Statistics," US Department of Health and Human Services, updated September 25, 2020, https://www.cdc.gov/ncbddd/autism/data.html.

3. Leo Kanner, "Autistic Disturbances of Affective Contact," *Nervous Child* 2 (1943): 217–50, http://simonsfoundation.s3.amazonaws.com/share/071207-leo-kanner-autistic-affective-contact.pdf.

4. Berend Verhoeff, "Autism in Flux: A History of the Concept from Leo Kanner to *DSM-5*," *History of Psychiatry* 24, no. 4 (December 2013): 442–58, https://doi.org /10.1177/0957154X13500584.

5. Verhoeff, "Autism in Flux."

6. Pauline Chaste and Marion Leboyer, "Autism Risk Factors: Genes, Environment, and Gene-Environment Interactions," *Dialogues in Clinical Neuroscience* 14, no. 3 (September 2012): 281–92, https://doi.org/10.31887/DCNS.2012.14.3/pchaste.

7. Judith H. Miles, "Autism Spectrum Disorders—a Genetics Review," *Genetics in Medicine* 13, no. 4 (April 2011): 278–94, https://doi.org/10.1097/GIM.0b013e3181ff67ba; Marlene B. Lauritsen and H. Ewald, "The Genetics of Autism," *Acta Psychiatrica Scandinavica* 103, no. 6 (June 2001): 411–27, https://doi.org/10.1034/j.1600-0447.2001.00086.x; Michael Waldman, Sean Nicholson, and Nodir Adilov, "Does Television Cause Autism?," (working paper 12632, National Bureau of Economic Research, October 2006), https://doi.org/10.3386/w12632.

8. Richard Horton, "A Statement by the Editors of *The Lancet*," *The Lancet* 363, no. 9411 (March 6, 2004): 820–21, https://doi.org/10.1016/S0140-6736(04)15699-7.

9. J. B. Barahona-Corrêa and Carlos N. Filipe, "A Concise History of Asperger Syndrome: The Short Reign of a Troublesome Diagnosis," *Frontiers in Psychology* 6, no. 2024 (January 25, 2016), https://doi.org/10.3389/fpsyg.2015.02024.

10. Greenberg, *Book of Woe*, 201–2.

11. Silberman, Steve. "The Geek Syndrome." *Wired*, December 1, 2001. https://www .wired.com/2001/12/aspergers/.

12. Pablo Neruda, *The Poetry of Pablo Neruda*, ed. Ilan Stavans (New York: Farrar, Straus and Giroux, 2003).

13. Marc-Antoine Crocq, "A History of Anxiety: From Hippocrates to DSM," *Dialogues in Clinical Neuroscience* 17, no. 3 (September 2015): 319–25, https://doi.org/10.31887 /DCNS.2015.17.3/macrocq.

14. Jitender Sareen *et al.*, "Anxiety Disorders and Risk for Suicidal Ideation and Suicide Attempts: A Population-Based Longitudinal Study of Adults," *Archives of General Psychiatry* 62, no. 11 (2005): 1249–57, https://doi.org/10.1001/archpsyc.62.11.1249; Arif Khan *et al.*, "Suicide Risk in Patients with Anxiety Disorders: A Meta-Analysis of the FDA Database," *Journal of Affective Disorders* 68, no. 1–2 (April 2002): 183–90, https://doi.org/10.1016/S0165-0327(01)00354-8.

15. Nicholas E. Calcaterra and James C. Barrow, "Classics in Chemical Neuroscience: Diazepam (Valium)," *ACS Chemical Neuroscience* 5, no. 4 (2014): 253–60, https://doi .org/10.1021/cn5000056.

16. Jonathan M. Metzl, "'Mother's Little Helper': The Crisis of Psychoanalysis and the Miltown Resolution," *Gender and History* 15, no. 2 (August 2003): 228–55, https://doi .org/10.1111/1468-0424.00300.

17. Robin Marantz Henig, "Valium's Contribution to Our New Normal," *New York Times*, September 29, 2012, https://www.nytimes.com/2012/09/30/sunday-review/valium -and-the-new-normal.html.

18. Jeannette Y. Wick, "The History of Benzodiazepines," *The Consultant Pharmacist* 28, no. 9 (September 2013): 538–48, https://doi.org/10.4140/TCP.n.2013.538.

19. Sidney Kessler, Joanna Hernik, and Dana-Nicoleta Lascu, "The Genesis of Robitussin's 'Ask Your Doctor' Campaign: The Prevalent Theme of Pharmaceutical Advertising for Four Decades," *Innovative Marketing* 9, no. 2 (2013 : 69–75.

20. Lisa M. Schwartz and Steven Woloshin, "Medical Marketing in the United States, 1997–2016," *JAMA* 321, no. 1 (2019): 80–96, https://doi.org/10.1001/jama.2018.19320.

21. Melanie Yergeau, "Circle Wars: Reshaping the Typical Autism Essay," *Disabilities Studies Quarterly* 30, no. 1 (2010), https://dsq-sds.org/article/view/1063/1222&gt.

6. Cracked

1. Mary G. Baker, Rajendra Kale, and Matthew Menken, "The Wall Between Neurology and Psychiatry," *BMJ* 324, no. 7352 (2002): 1468–69, https://doi.org/10.1136/bmj.324.7352.1468.

2. American Psychiatric Association, *Diagnostic and Statistical Manual of Mental Disorders*, 3rd ed. *(DSM-III)* (Washington, DC: American Psychiatric Association, 1980).

3. William E. Pelham Jr. *et al.*, "Teacher Ratings of DSM-III-R Symptoms for the Disruptive Behavior Disorders," *Journal of the American Academy of Child and Adolescent Psychiatry* 31, no. 2 (March 1992): 210–18, https://doi.org/10.1097/00004583-199203000-00006.

4. Adrian Angold and E. Jane Costello, "Toward Establishing an Empirical Basis for the Diagnosis of Oppositional Defiant Disorder," *Journal of the American Academy of Child and Adolescent Psychiatry* 35, no. 9 (September 1996): 1205–12, https://doi.org/10.1097/00004583-199609000-00018.

5. Benjamin B. Lahey *et al.*, "DSM-IV Field Trials for Oppositional Defiant Disorder and Conduct Disorder in Children and Adolescents," *American Journal of Psychiatry* 151, no. 8 (August 1994): 1163–71, https://doi.org/10.1176/ajp.151.8.1163.

6. Substance Abuse and Mental Health Services Administration, "Table 18: DSM-IV to DSM-5 Oppositional Defiant Disorder Comparison," in *DSM-5 Changes: Implications for Child Serious Emotional Disturbance* (Rockville, MD: Substance Abuse and Mental Health Services Administration, June 2016), https://www.ncbi.nlm.nih.gov/books/NBK519712/table/ch3.t14.

7. Sarah Maria Birkle *et al.*, "Disruptive Affektregulations Störung: Eine Umstrittene Neue Diagnose im DSM-5 [Disruptive Mood Dysregulation Disorder: A Controversial New Diagnostic Entity in the DSM-5]," *Zeitschrift für Kinder- und Jugendpsychiatrie und Psychotherapie* 45, no. 2 (March 2017): 98–103, https://doi.org/10.1024/1422-4917/a000496.

8. Dustin A. Pardini and Paula J. Fite, "Symptoms of Conduct Disorder, Oppositional Defiant Disorder, Attention-Deficit/Hyperactivity Disorder, and Callous-Unemotional Traits as Unique Predictors of Psychosocial Maladjustment in Boys: Advancing an Evidence Base for *DSM-V*," *Journal of the American Academy of Child and Adolescent Psychiatry* 49, no. 11 (November 2010): 1134–44, https://doi.org/10.1016%2Fj.jaac.2010.07.010.

9. Joseph Day, "The Effect of Race on the Diagnosis of Oppositional Defiant Disorder," Education Resources Information Center, November 14, 2002, https://eric.ed.gov/?id=ED470718.

10. Cheryl B. McNeil, Laura C. Capage, and Gwendolyn M. Bennett, "Cultural Issues in the Treatment of Young African American Children Diagnosed with Disruptive Behavior Disorders," *Journal of Pediatric Psychology* 27, no. 4 (June 2002): 339–50, https://doi.org/10.1093/jpepsy/27.4.339; Matthew C. Fadus *et al.*, "Unconscious Bias and the Diagnosis of Disruptive Behavior Disorders and ADHD in African American and Hispanic Youth," *Academic Psychiatry* 44 (2020): 95–102, https://doi.org/10.1007/s40596-019-01127-6; Kess L. Ballentine, "Understanding Racial Differences in Diagnosing ODD Versus ADHD Using Critical Race Theory," *Families in Society:*

The Journal of Contemporary Social Services 100, no. 3 (July 2019): 282–92, https://doi.org/10.1177/1044389419842765; June Liang, Brittany E. Matheson, and Jennifer M. Douglas, "Mental Health Diagnostic Considerations in Racial/Ethnic Minority Youth," *Journal of Child and Family Studies* 25, no. 6 (2016): 1926–40, https://doi.org/10.1007/s10826-015-0351-z.

11. David R. Williams and Michelle Harris-Reid, "Race and Mental Health: Emerging Patterns and Promising Approaches," in *A Handbook for the Study of Mental Health: Social Contexts, Theories, and Systems*, ed. A. V. Horwitz and T. L. Scheid (Cambridge: Cambridge University Press, 1999), 295–314.

12. David S. Mandell *et al.*, "Disparities in Diagnoses Received Prior to a Diagnosis of Autism Spectrum Disorder," *Journal of Autism and Developmental Disorders* 37, no. 9 (October 2007): 1795–802, https://doi.org/10.1007/s10803-006-0314-8.

13. Robert C. Schwartz and David M. Blankenship, "Racial Disparities in Psychotic Disorder Diagnosis: A Review of Empirical Literature," *World Journal of Psychiatry* 4, no. 4 (December 2014): 133–40, https://doi.org/10.5498/wjp.v4.i4.133.

14. Harrington, *Mind Fixers*, 206; Georgia State University, "Racial, Ethnic Differences Found in Psychiatric Diagnoses, Treatment, according to Researchers," ScienceDaily, May 18, 2016, https://www.sciencedaily.com/releases/2016/05/160518094721.htm; Arnold Barnes, "Race, Schizophrenia, and Admission to State Psychiatric Hospitals," *Administration and Policy in Mental Health and Mental Health Services Research* 31 (2004): 241–52, https://doi.org/10.1023/B:APIH.0000018832.73673.54.

15. Karen J. Coleman *et al.*, "Racial-Ethnic Differences in Psychiatric Diagnoses and Treatment across 11 Health Care Systems in the Mental Health Research Network," *Psychiatric Services* 67, no. 7 (July 2016): 749–57, https://doi.org/10.1176/appi.ps.201500217; "Mental Health Disparities: Diverse Populations," American Psychiatric Association, https://www.psychiatry.org/psychiatrists/cultural-competency/education/mental-health-facts.

16. Coleman *et al.*, "Racial-Ethnic Differences in Psychiatric Diagnoses."

17. Joshua Breslau *et al.*, "Lifetime Risk and Persistence of Psychiatric Disorders across Ethnic Groups in the United States," *Psychological Medicine* 35, no. 3 (March 2005): 317–27, https://doi.org/10.1017/s0033291704003514; Thomas G. McGuire and Jeanne Miranda, "New Evidence Regarding Racial and Ethnic Disparities in Mental Health: Policy Implications," *Health Affairs* 27, no. 2 (March/April 2008): 393–403, https://doi.org/10.1377/hlthaff.27.2.393.

18. John Elflein, "Percentage of U.S. Americans without Health Insurance by Ethnicity 2010–2020," Statista, April 15, 2021, https://www.statista.com/statistics/200970/percentage-of-americans-without-health-insurance-by-race-ethnicity/; McGuire and Miranda, "New Evidence Regarding Racial and Ethnic Disparities"; Oanh L. Meyer and Nolan Zane, "The Influence of Race and Ethnicity in Clients' Experiences of Mental Health Treatment," *Journal of Community Psychology* 41, no. 7 (September 2013): 884–901, https://doi.org/10.1002/jcop.21580.

19. Rodney A. Samaan, "The Influences of Race, Ethnicity, and Poverty on the Mental Health of Children," *Journal of Health Care for the Poor and Underserved* 11, no. 1 (February 2000): 100–10, https://doi.org/10.1353/hpu.2010.0557; Faye A. Gary, "Stigma: Barrier to Mental Health Care Among Ethnic Minorities," *Issues in Mental Health Nursing* 26, no. 10 (2005): 979–99, https://doi.org/10.1080/01612840500280638; "Black/African American," National Alliance on Mental Illness, accessed July 2020, https://www.nami.org/Your-Journey/Identity-and-Cultural-Dimensions/Black-African

-American; "Hispanic/Latinx," National Alliance on Mental Illness, accessed July 2020, https://www.nami.org/Your-Journey/Identity-and-Cultural-Dimensions/Latinx -Hispanic; "Mental Health Disparities: Diverse Populations."

20. Individuals with Disabilities Education Act, Section 300.8(c)(4), US Department of Education (May 2, 2017), https://sites.ed.gov/idea/regs/b/a/300.8/c/4.

21. Kelly R. Tan, Uwe Rudolph, and Christian Lüscher, "Hooked on Benzodiazepines: GABA$_A$ Receptor Subtypes and Addiction," *Trends in Neurosciences* 34, no. 4 (April 2011): 188–97, https://dx.doi.org/10.1016%2Fj.tins.2011.01.004; Glen O. Gabbard, *Gabbard's Treatments of Psychiatric Disorders* (Washington, DC: American Psychiatric Association Publishing, 2007).

22. Tan, Rudolph, and Lüscher, "Hooked on Benzodiazepines"; NIDA Notes Staff, "Well-Known Mechanism Underlies Benzodiazepines' Addictive Properties," National Institute on Drug Abuse, April 19, 2012, https://archives.drugabuse.gov/news-events /nida-notes/2012/04/well-known-mechanism-underlies-benzodiazepines-addictive -properties.

23. James E. Sabin and Norman Daniels, "Determining 'Medical Necessity' in Mental Health Practice," *The Hastings Center Report* 24, no. 6 (November–December 1994): 5–13, https://www.jstor.org/stable/3563458.

24. Owen Whooley, "Diagnostic Ambivalence: Psychiatric Workarounds and the Diagnostic and Statistical Manual of Mental Disorders," *Sociology of Health and Illness* 32, no. 3 (March 2010): 452–69, https://doi.org/10.1111/j.1467-9566.2010.01230.x.

25. Greenberg, *Book of Woe*, 67–68.

26. The Editors, "Clinical Trials Have Far Too Little Racial and Ethnic Diversity," *Scientific American*, September 1, 2008, https://www.scientificamerican.com/article /clinical-trials-have-far-too-little-racial-and-ethnic-diversity/.

7. Doctor's Orders

1. Jonathan S. Abramowitz and Ryan J. Jacoby, "Obsessive-Compulsive Disorder in the *DSM-5*," *Clinical Psychology: Science and Practice* 21, no. 3 (2014): 221–35, https:// psycnet.apa.org/doi/10.1111/cpsp.12076; Kimberly Glazier, Matt Swing, and Lata K. McGinn, "Half of Obsessive-Compulsive Disorder Cases Misdiagnosed," *The Journal of Clinical Psychiatry* 76, no. 6 (2015): e761–67, https://doi.org/10.4088/jcp.14m09110.

2. Antony Barnett, "Trouble in Transcendental Paradise as Murder Rocks the Maharishi University," *The Guardian*, May 1, 2004, https://www.theguardian.com/world/2004 /may/02/usa.theobserver.

3. Assen Jablensky, "The Diagnostic Concept of Schizophrenia: Its History, Evolution, and Future Prospects," *Dialogues in Clinical Neuroscience* 12, no. 3 (September 2010): 271–87, https://doi.org/10.31887/DCNS.2010.12.3/ajablensky; Mahendra T. Bhati, "Defining Psychosis: The Evolution of DSM-5 Schizophrenia Spectrum Disorders," *Current Psychiatry Reports* 15, no. 11 (November 2013): 409, https://doi.org/10.1007 /s11920-013-0409-9.

4. Andrew Moskowitz and Gerhard Heim, "Eugen Bleuler's *Dementia Praecox or the Group of Schizophrenias* (1911): A Centenary Appreciation and Reconsideration," *Schizophrenia Bulletin* 37, no. 3 (May 2011): 471–79, https://doi.org/10.1093/schbul /sbr016.

5. Harrington, *Mind Fixers*, 139.

6. Bhati, "Defining Psychosis."

7. A. Ban Thomas, "Evolution of Diagnostic Criteria in Psychoses," *Dialogues in*

Clinical Neuroscience 3, no. 4 (December 2001): 257–63, https://doi.org/10.31887 /DCNS.2001.3.4/abthomas.

8. Johns Hopkins Medicine, "Study Suggests Overdiagnosis of Schizophrenia," ScienceDaily, April 22, 2019, https://www.sciencedaily.com/releases/2019/04/19042209 0842.htm; Jennifer Bartlett, "Childhood-Onset Schizophrenia: What Do We Really Know?," *Health Psychology and Behavioral Medicine* 2, no. 1 (2014): 735–47, https:// doi.org/10.1080/21642850.2014.927738.

9. Estate of Butler v. Maharishi University of Management, 589 F. Supp. 2d 1150 (S.D. Iowa 2008), https://law.justia.com/cases/federal/district-courts/FSupp2/589/1150/1870047/.

10. Krzysztof Dyga and Radosław Stupak, "Meditation and Psychosis: Trigger or Cure?," *Archives of Psychiatry and Psychotherapy* 3 (2015): 48–58, https://doi.org/10.12740 /APP/58976; P. Sharma et al., "Meditation—a Two Edged Sword for Psychosis: A Case Report," Irish Journal of Psychological Medicine 33, no. 4 (2016): 247–49, https://doi .org/10.1017/ipm.2015.73.

11. Estate of Butler v. Maharishi University of Management.

12. Joseph Weber, *Transcendental Meditation in America: How a New Age Movement Remade a Small Town in Iowa* (Iowa City: University of Iowa Press, 2014).

13. Robert Whitaker, *Anatomy of an Epidemic: Magic Bullets, Psychiatric Drugs, and the Astonishing Rise of Mental Illness in America* (New York: Crown Archetype, 2010), 115, Kindle.

14. Matt Ford, "America's Largest Mental Hospital Is a Jail," *The Atlantic*, June 8, 2015, https://www.theatlantic.com/politics/archive/2015/06/americas-largest-mental-hospital -is-a-jail/395012/.

15. Heather Stuart, "Violence and Mental Illness: An Overview," *World Psychiatry* 2, no. 2 (June 2003): 121–24, https://www.ncbi.nlm.nih.gov/pmc/articles/PMC1525086/; Mohit Varshney *et al.*, "Violence and Mental Illness: What Is the True Story?," *Journal of Epidemiology and Community Health* 70, no. 3 (March 2016): 223–25, http://dx.doi .org/10.1136/jech-2015-205546; Marie E. Rueve and Randon S. Welton, "Violence and Mental Illness," *Psychiatry* 5, no. 5 (May 2008): 34–48, https://www.ncbi.nlm.nih.gov/pmc /articles/PMC2686644/.

16. "Mental Health Myths and Facts," MentalHealth.gov, US Department of Health and Human Services, accessed, July 2020, https://www.mentalhealth.gov/basics/mental -health-myths-facts.

17. Rob Whitley, "The Antipsychiatry Movement: Dead, Diminishing, or Developing?," *Psychiatric Services* 63, no. 10 (October 2012): 1039–41, https://doi.org/10.1176/appi .ps.201100484.

18. Thomas J. Scheff, *Being Mentally Ill: A Sociological Study* (New York: Routledge, 1999).

19. Ronald David Laing, *The Politics of Experience* (New York: Pantheon, 1983).

20. D. L. Rosenhan, "On Being Sane in Insane Places," *Science* 179, no. 4070 (January 19, 1973): 250–58, https://doi.org/10.1126/science.179.4070.250.

21. Susannah Cahalan, The Great Pretender: *The Undercover Mission That Changed Our Understanding of Madness* (New York: Grand Central Publishing, 2019).

22. "Schizophrenia," National Institute of Mental Health, last revised May 2020, https:// www.nimh.nih.gov/health/topics/schizophrenia/index.shtml; Alan Breier *et al.*, "National Institute of Mental Health Longitudinal Study of Chronic Schizophrenia: Prognosis and Predictors of Outcome," *Archives of General Psychiatry* 48, no. 3 (1991): 239–46, https://doi.org/10.1001/archpsyc.1991.01810270051007.

23. Robin M. Murray, "Mistakes I Have Made in My Research Career," *Schizophrenia Bulletin* 43, no. 2 (March 2017): 253–56, https://doi.org/10.1093/schbul/sbw165; Jim

van Os, "'Schizophrenia' Does Not Exist," *BMJ* 352 (2016), https://doi.org/10.1136/bmj.i375; Tyrone D. Cannon *et al.*, "The Genetic Epidemiology of Schizophrenia in a Finnish Twin Cohort," *Archives of General Psychiatry* 55, no. 1 (1998): 67–74, https://doi.org/10.1001/archpsyc.55.1.67; Harvard Health Publishing, "Schizophrenia," Harvard Medical School, February 1, 2019, https://www.health.harvard.edu/a_to_z/schizophrenia-a-to-z; Schizophrenia Working Group of the Psychiatric Genomics Consortium, "Biological Insights from 108 Schizophrenia-Associated Genetic Loci," *Nature* 511 (2014): 421–27, https://doi.org/10.1038/nature13595.

24. Godfrey D. Pearlson and Laura Marsh, "Structural Brain Imaging in Schizophrenia: A Selective Review," *Biological Psychiatry* 46 (1999): 627–49.

25. Szasz, *The Myth of Mental Illness*.

26. Judith Warner, "The Denial of Mental Illness Is Alive and Well," *Time*, September 14, 2012, https://ideas.time.com/2012/09/14/the-denial-of-mental-illness-is-alive-and-well/.

8. Treatment/Options

1. Scott Gottlieb, "Methylphenidate Works by Increasing Dopamine Levels," *BMJ (Clinical Research Edition)* 322, no. 7281 (February 2001): 259, https://www.bmj.com/content/322/7281/259.3.full.

2. University of Wisconsin–Madison, "How Ritalin Works in Brain to Boost Cognition, Focus Attention," ScienceDaily, June 25, 2008, https://www.sciencedaily.com/releases/2008/06/080624115956.htm.

3. Lily Hechtman *et al.*, "Diagnosing ADHD in Adults: Limitations to DSM-IV and DSM-V Proposals and Challenges Ahead," *Neuropsychiatry* 1, no. 6 (December 2011): 579–90, https://www.researchgate.net/publication/274667077_Diagnosing_ADHD_in__adults_limitations_to_DSM-IV_and_DSM-V_proposals_and_challenges_ahead; Frances, *Saving Normal*, 183.

4. Dusan Kolar *et al.*, "Treatment of Adults with Attention-Deficit/Hyperactivity Disorder," *Neuropsychiatric Disease and Treatment* 4, no. 2 (April 2008): 389–403, https://doi.org/10.2147/ndt.s6985.

5. Joanna Moncrieff and Sami Timimi, "Critical Analysis of the Concept of Adult Attention-Deficit Hyperactivity Disorder," *The Psychiatrist* 35, no. 9 (2011): 334–38, https://doi.org/10.1192/pb.bp.110.033423.

6. Nicola Morant et al., "The Least Worst Option: User Experiences of Antipsychotic Medication and Lack of Involvement in Medication Decisions in a UK Community Sample," *Journal of Mental Health* 27, no. 4 (2017): 322–28, https://doi.org/10.1080/09638237.2017.1370637; Denise Mann, "What to Do When Your Depression Treatment Isn't Working," WebMD, October 1, 2021, https://www.webmd.com/depression/features/treatment-not-working.

7. H. P. Chin *et al.*, "Psychiatric Training in Primary Care Medicine Residency Programs: A National Survey," *Psychosomatics* 41, no. 5 (September–October 2000): 412–17, https://doi.org/10.1176/appi.psy.41.5.412.

8. Robert C. Smith, "Educating Trainees About Common Mental Health Problems in Primary Care: A (Not So) Modest Proposal," *Academic Medicine* 86, no. 11 (November 2011): e16, https://doi.org/10.1097/ACM.0b013e3182308dc8.

9. Smith, "Educating Trainees About Common Mental Health Problems."

10. Hoyle Leigh, Deborah Stewart, and Ronna R. Mallios, "Mental Health and Psychiatry Training in Primary Care Residency Programs: Part I. Who Teaches, Where, When

and How Satisfied?," *General Hospital Psychiatry* 28, no. 3 (May–June 2006): 189–94, https://doi.org/10.1016/j.genhosppsych.2005.10.003.

11. Robert C. Smith *et al.*, "Addressing Mental Health Issues in Primary Care: An Initial Curriculum for Medical Residents," *Patient Education and Counseling* 94, no. 1 (January 2014): 33–42, http://dx.doi.org/10.1016/j.pec.2013.09.010.

12. Sharon Sanders *et al.*, "A Review of Changes to the Attention Deficit/Hyperactivity Disorder Age of Onset Criterion Using the Checklist for Modifying Disease Definitions," *BMC Psychiatry* 19 (2019): 357, https://doi.org/10.1186/s12888-019-2337-7; Jeffery N. Epstein and Richard E. A. Loren, "Changes in the Definition of ADHD in DSM-5: Subtle but Important," *Neuropsychiatry* 3, no. 5 (October 2013): 455–58, https://www.ncbi.nlm.nih.gov/pmc/articles/PMC3955126/.

13. Alicia Holland, "The Surprising History of the Slash," eType, August 27, 2017, http://etype.com/blog/surprising-history-slash/.

14. Christine B. Phillips, "Medicine Goes to School, Teachers as Sickness Brokers for ADHD," *PLoS Medicine* 3, no. 4 (April 2006): e182, https://doi.org/10.1371/journal.pmed.0030182.

15. Anna Baumgaertel, Mark L. Wolraich, and Mary Dietrich, "Comparison of Diagnostic Criteria for Attention Deficit Disorders in a German Elementary School Sample," *Journal of the American Academy of Child and Adolescent Psychiatry* 34, no. 5 (May 1995): 629–38, https://doi.org/10.1097/00004583-199505000-00015.

16. Sanders et al., "A Review of Changes to the Attention Deficit/Hyperactivity Disorder Age of Onset Criterion."

17. Epstein and Loren, "Changes in the Definition of ADHD in DSM-5."

18. Karen Thomas, "Back to School for ADHD Drugs," *USA Today*, August 28, 2001, http://usatoday30.usatoday.com/life/2001-08-28-adhd.htm.

19. Carrie S. Martin, "DDMAC Targets ADHD Products—FDA Issues Five Warning Letters on the Same Day," FDA Law Blog, Hyman, Phelps and McNamara PC, September 29, 2008, https://www.thefdalawblog.com/2008/09/ddmac-targets-a/.

20. Marnie Klein, "Masked Marketing: Pharmaceutical Company Funding of ADHD Patient Advocacy Groups," The Hastings Center, June 29, 2017, https://www.thehastingscenter.org/masked-marketing-pharmaceutical-company-funding-adhd-patient-advocacy-groups/.

21. Alan Schwarz, "The Selling of Attention Deficit Disorder," *New York Times*, December 14, 2013, https://www.nytimes.com/2013/12/15/health/the-selling-of-attention-deficit-disorder.html.

22. Jessica Mitchell and John Read, "Attention-Deficit Hyperactivity Disorder, Drug Companies and the Internet," *Clinical Child Psychology and Psychiatry* 17, no. 1 (2011): 121–39, https://doi.org/10.1177/1359104510396432.

23. Matthew S. McCoy *et al.*, "Conflicts of Interest for Patient-Advocacy Organizations," *The New England Journal of Medicine* 376, no. 9 (2017): 880–85, https://doi.org/10.1056/NEJMsr1610625; Phillips, "Medicine Goes to School"; "For Educators, Overview," Children and Adults with Attention-Deficit/Hyperactivity Disorder (CHADD), accessed July 2020, https://chadd.org/for-educators/overview/.

24. "ADHD. The Struggle Is Real," ADHD Adulthood, Takeda Pharmaceutical, 2020, https://www.adhdadulthood.com/.

25. Richard L. Morrow *et al.*, "Influence of Relative Age on Diagnosis and Treatment of Attention-Deficit/Hyperactivity Disorder in Children," *Canadian Medical Association Journal* 184, no. 7 (April 17, 2012): 755–62, https://doi.org/10.1503

/cmaj.111619; D. J. Safer, J. M. Zito, and E. M. Fine, "Increased Methylphenidate Usage for Attention Deficit Disorder in the 1990s," *Pediatrics* 98, no. 6 Part 1 (December 1996): 1084–88, https://pubmed.ncbi.nlm.nih.gov/8951257/; Daniel Goleman, "Scientist at Work: Allen J. Frances; Revamping Psychiatrists' Bible," *New York Times*, April 19, 1994, https://www.nytimes.com/1994/04/19/science/scientist-at-work-allen -j-frances-revamping-psychiatrists-bible.html; Benedict Carey, "Keith Conners, Psychologist Who Set Standard for Diagnosing A.D.H.D., Dies at 84," *New York Times*, July 13, 2017, https://www.nytimes.com/2017/07/13/health/keith-conners-deadpsych ologist-adhd-diagnosing.html; Alan Schwarz, "The Selling of Attention Deficit Disorder," *New York Times*, December 14, 2013, https://www.nytimes.com/2013/12/15 /health/the-selling-of-attention-deficit-disorder.html.

26. Frances, *Saving Normal*, 138.

27. D. H. Shapiro Jr., "Adverse Effects of Meditation: A Preliminary Investigation of Long-Term Meditators," *International Journal of Psychosomatic Research* 39, no. 1–4 (1992): 62–67, https://pubmed.ncbi.nlm.nih.gov/1428622/.

28. Tim Lomas *et al.*, "A Qualitative Analysis of Experiential Challenges Associated with Meditation Practice," *Mindfulness* 6, no. 4 (August 2015): 848–60, https://doi .org/10.1007/s12671-014-0329-8.

29. Ausiàs Cebolla *et al.*, "Unwanted Effects: Is There a Negative Side of Meditation? A Multicentre Survey," *PLoS One* 12, no. 9 (2017): e0183137, https://doi.org/10.1371 /journal.pone.0183137.

30. Azmeh Shahid *et al.*, "Hamilton Rating Scale for Depression (HAM-D)," in *STOP, THAT and One Hundred Other Sleep Scales*, ed. Azmeh Shahid *et al.* (Secaucus, NJ: Springer Science and Business Media, 2012), 187–90.

31. Henri-Frédéric Amiel, *Amiel's Journal* (Project Gutenberg, July 2005), https://www .gutenberg.org/files/8545/8545-h/8545-h.htm.

32. Norman Sartorious, "Comorbidity of Mental and Physical Diseases: A Main Challenge for Medicine of the 21st Century," *Shanghai Archives of Psychiatry* 25, no. 2 (April 2013): 68–69, https://www.ncbi.nlm.nih.gov/pmc/articles/PMC4054544/; Hanna M. van Loo and Jan-Willem Romeijn, "Psychiatric Comorbidity: Fact or Artifact?," *Theoretical Medicine and Bioethics* 36, no. 1 (2015): 41–60, https://dx.doi.org/10.1007 %2Fs11017-015-9321-0.

33. Ronald C. Kessler *et al.*, "Prevalence, Severity, and Comorbidity of 12-Month DSM-IV Disorders in the National Comorbidity Survey Replication," *Archives of General Psychiatry* 62, no. 6 (2005): 617–27, https://doi.org/10.1001/archpsyc.62.6.617.

34. Oleguer Plana-Ripoll *et al.*, "Exploring Comorbidity within Mental Disorders among a Danish National Population," *JAMA Psychiatry* 76, no. 3 (March 2019): 259–70, https://doi.org/10.1001/jamapsychiatry.2018.3658.

35. Van Loo and Romeijn, "Psychiatric Comorbidity: Fact or Artifact?"

36. R. L. Spitzer and P. T. Wilson, "Section 7: A Guide to the New Nomenclature," in American Psychiatric Association, *Diagnostic and Statistical Manual of Mental Disorders*, 2nd ed. (DSM-II) (Washington, DC: American Psychiatric Association, 1968), 122–23; Horwitz, *DSM*, 42.

37. David W. Goodman and Michael E. Thase, "Recognizing ADHD in Adults with Comorbid Mood Disorders: Implications for Identification and Management," *Postgraduate Medicine* 121, no. 5 (September 2009): 31–41, https://doi.org/10.3810/pgm .2009.09.2049.

9. Becoming Bipolar

1. Franklin E. Zimring and Gordon Hawkins, "Crime, Justice, and the Savings and Loan Crisis," *Crime and Justice* 18 (1993): 247–92, https://www.jstor.org/stable/1147658.
2. Nina Siegal, "What Ailed van Gogh? Doctors Weigh In," *New York Times*, September 15, 2016, https://www.nytimes.com/2016/09/16/arts/design/vincent-van-gogh-doctors-historians-weigh-in-amsterdam.html; "Health of Vincent van Gogh," Wikipedia, last modified January 14, 2021, https://en.wikipedia.org/wiki/Health_of_Vincent_van_Gogh.
3. Dara Mohammadi, "Nancy C. Andreasen: Creativity and Mental Illness," *The Lancet* 4, no. 3 (March 2017): 192, https://doi.org/10.1016/S2215-0366(17)30013-5.
4. N. J. C. Andreasen and Arthur Canter, "The Creative Writer: Psychiatric Symptoms and Family History," *Comprehensive Psychiatry* 15, no. 2 (March–April 1974): 123–31, https://doi.org/10.1016/0010-440X(74)90028-5.
5. Mohammadi, "Nancy C. Andreasen."
6. Kay Redfield Jamison, "Mood Disorders and Patterns of Creativity in British Writers and Artists," *Psychiatry* 52, no. 2 (1989): 125–34, https://doi.org/10.1080/00332747.1989.11024436.
7. Kay Redfield Jamison, *Touched with Fire: Manic-Depressive Illness and the Artistic Temperament* (New York: Free Press, 1993), 17, Kindle.
8. Kay Redfield Jamison, *An Unquiet Mind: A Memoir of Moods and Madness* (New York: Knopf Doubleday Publishing Group, 1995), Kindle.
9. Claudia Kalb, *Andy Warhol Was a Hoarder: Inside the Minds of History's Great Personalities* (New York: Disney Book Group, 2016), 18, Kindle.
10. Colin Bird, "Do You Know What This Symbol Means?," Cars.com, June 5, 2017, https://www.cars.com/articles/do-you-know-what-this-symbol-means-1420663197854/.
11. Rose Eveleth, "The History of the Exclamation Point," *Smithsonian Magazine*, August 9, 2012, https://www.smithsonianmag.com/smart-news/the-history-of-the-exclamation-point-16445416/.
12. Geoff Nunberg, "After Years of Restraint, a Linguist Says 'Yes!' to the Exclamation Point," June 13, 2017, in *Fresh Air*, produced by NPR, radio broadcast, MP3 audio, 8:39, https://www.npr.org/2017/06/08/532148705/after-years-of-restraint-a-linguist-says-yes-to-the-exclamation-point.
13. Bird, "Do You Know What This Symbol Means?"; Carol Waseleski, "Gender and the Use of Exclamation Points in Computer-Mediated Communication: An Analysis of Exclamations Posted to Two Electronic Discussion Lists," *Journal of Computer-Mediated Communication* 11, no. 4 (July 2006): 1012–24, https://doi.org/10.1111/j.1083-6101.2006.00305.x.
14. Johns Hopkins Medicine, "Mental Health Disorder Statistics," John Hopkins Medicine, 2019, https://www.hopkinsmedicine.org/health/wellness-and-prevention/mental-health-disorder-statistics; "You Are Not Alone," National Alliance on Mental Illness, https://www.nami.org/NAMI/media/NAMI-Media/Infographics/NAMI_YouAreNotAlone_2020_FINAL.pdf.
15. Liza H. Gold, "DSM-5 and the Assessment of Functioning: The World Health Organization Disability Assessment Schedule 2.0 (WHODAS 2.0)," *Journal of the American Academy of Psychiatry and the Law Online* 42, no. 2 (June 2014): 173–81, http://jaapl.org/content/42/2/173#sec-9.
16. National Institute of Mental Health, "Mental Illness," updated January 2021, https://www.nimh.nih.gov/health/statistics/mental-illness.shtml.

17. "Mental Illness," National Institute of Mental Health.
18. Frederick Cassidy *et al.*, "A Factor Analysis of the Signs and Symptoms of Mania," *Archives of General Psychiatry* 55, no. 1 (1998): 27–32, https://doi.org/10.1001/arch psyc.55.1.27.
19. Brittany L. Mason, E. Sherwood Brown, and Paul E. Croarkin, "Historical Underpinnings of Bipolar Disorder Diagnostic Criteria," *Behavioral Sciences* 6, no. 3 (September 2016): 14, https://dx.doi.org/10.3390%2Fbs6030014.
20. Jules Angst, "Historical Aspects of the Dichotomy Between Manic–Depressive Disorders and Schizophrenia," *Schizophrenia Research* 57, no. 1 (September 2002): 5–13, https://doi.org/10.1016/S0920-9964(02)00328-6.
21. Mason, Brown, and Croarkin, "Historical Underpinnings."
22. Michael J. Ostacher, Mark A. Frye, and Trisha Suppes, "Bipolar Disorders in DSM-5: Changes and Implications for Clinical Research," in *Bipolar Disorders: Basic Mechanisms and Therapeutic Implications*, ed. Jair C. Soares (Cambridge: Cambridge University Press, 2016), 1–7; American Psychiatric Association, *DSM-5*.
23. Janet Lee and Karen L. Swartz, "Bipolar I Disorder," *John Hopkins Psychiatry Guide*, updated October 29, 2017, https://www.hopkinsguides.com/hopkins/view/Johns_Hop kins_Psychiatry_Guide/787045/all/Bipolar_I_Disorder.
24. Smitha Bhandari, "What Are Hypomania and Mania in Bipolar Disorder?," WebMD, September 12, 2020, https://www.webmd.com/bipolar-disorder/guide/hypomania -mania -symptoms.
25. Franco Benazzi and Zoltan Rihmer, "Sensitivity and Specificity of DSM-IV Atypical Features for Bipolar II Disorder Diagnosis," Psychiatry Research 93, no. 3 (April 2000): 257–62, https://doi.org/10.1016/S0165-1781(00)00121-9.

10. When the Happy Pill Ends

1. James Roland, "Bipolar 1 Disorder and Bipolar 2 Disorder: What Are the Differences?," Healthline, updated January 10, 2019, https://www.healthline.com/health /bipolar-disorder/bipolar-1-vs-bipolar-2; Matthew Hoffman, "Bipolar II Disorder," WebMD, April 14, 2020, https://www.webmd.com/bipolar-disorder/guide/bipolar-2 -disorder.
2. Daniel B. Block, "Bipolar Disorder," Verywell Mind, November 2, 2020, https://www .verywellmind.com/bipolar-disorder-4157274.
3. Lauren M. Weinstock *et al.*, "Differential Item Functioning of DSM-IV Depressive Symptoms in Individuals with a History of Mania Versus Those without: An Item Response Theory Analysis," *Bipolar Disorders* 11, no. 3 (May 2009): 289–97, https://doi .org/10.1111/j.1399-5618.2009.00681.x.
4. Zubin Bhagwagar and Guy M. Goodwin, "Bipolar-Spectrum Disorders: An Epidemic Unseen, Invisible or Unreal?," *Advances in Psychiatric Treatment* 10, no. 1 (January 2004): 1–3, https://doi.org/10.1192/apt.10.1.1; Maria Faurholt-Jepsen *et al.*, "Differences in Mood Instability in Patients with Bipolar Disorder Type I and II: A Smartphone-Based Study," *International Journal of Bipolar Disorders* 7 (2019): article 5, https://doi .org/10.1186/s40345-019-0141-4; Frances, *Saving Normal*, 150.
5. Franco Benazzi, "Factor Structure of Recalled DSM-IV Hypomanic Symptoms of Bipolar II Disorder," *Comprehensive Psychiatry* 45, no. 6 (November–December 2004): 441–46, https://doi.org/10.1016/j.comppsych.2004.07.004.
6. Franco Benazzi, "Depressive Mixed States: Unipolar and Bipolar II," *European Archives of Psychiatry and Clinical Neuroscience* 250 (2000): 249–53, https://doi.org

/10.1007/s004060070014; Jules Angst, "The Emerging Epidemiology of Hypomania and Bipolar II Disorder," *Journal of Affective Disorders* 50, no. 2–3 (September 1998): 143–51, https://doi.org/10.1016/S0165-0327(98)00142-6; Frances, *Saving Normal*, 149.

7. David L. Dunner, "Clinical Consequences of Under-Recognized Bipolar Spectrum Disorder," *Bipolar Disorders* 5, no. 6 (December 2003): 456–63, https://doi.org/10.1046/j.1399-5618.2003.00073.x; Harrington, *Mind Fixers*, 244.

8. Hagop S. Akiskal and Olavo Pinto, "The Evolving Bipolar Spectrum: Prototypes I, II, III, and IV," *Psychiatric Clinics of North America* 22, no. 3 (September 1999): 517–34, https://doi.org/10.1016/S0193-953X(05)70093-9.

9. Dunner, "Clinical Consequences of Under-Recognized Bipolar Spectrum Disorder."

10. American Psychiatric Association, *Diagnostic and Statistical Manual of Mental Disorders*, 4th ed. (*DSM-IV*) (Washington, DC: American Psychiatric Association, 1994), 365.

11. Ross J. Baldessarini, "A Plea for Integrity of the Bipolar Disorder Concept," *Bipolar Disorders* 2, no. 1 (March 2000): 3–7, https://doi.org/10.1034/j.1399-5618.2000.020102.x.

12. Mark Zimmerman *et al.*, "Is Bipolar Disorder Overdiagnosed?," *Journal of Clinical Psychiatry* 69, no. 6 (June 2008): 935–40, https://doi.org/10.4088/jcp.v69n0608.

13. Allen Frances (@AllenFrancesMD), "Before DSM-IV #bipolardisorder was under-diagnosed. We added Bipolar-II to protect patients against antidepressant switches & rapid cycling. Drug cos sold BP2 . . .," Twitter, June 6, 2019, https://twitter.com/AllenFrancesMD/status/1136583524801101825.

14. Frances, *Saving Normal*, 75.

15. Frances, *Saving Normal*, 75.

16. Frances, *Saving Normal*, 73.

17. Frances, *Saving Normal*, 73.

18. Frances, *Saving Normal*, 75.

19. Frances, *Saving Normal*, 73.

20. Allen Frances *et al.*, *DSM-IV Guidebook* (Washington, DC: American Psychiatric Association, 1995), https://psycnet.apa.org/record/1995-97831-000.

21. Frances, *Saving Normal*, 73.

22. Frances, *Saving Normal*, 76.

23. Frances, *Saving Normal*, 69.

24. Frances, *Saving Normal*, 75.

25. Lilly Shanahan *et al.*, "Does Despair Really Kill? A Roadmap for an Evidence-Based Answer," *American Journal of Public Health* 109, no. 6 (June 2019): 854–58, https://dx.doi.org/10.2105%2FAJPH.2019.305016.

26. Blake Dodge, "What Are So-Called Deaths of Despair? Experts Say They're on the Rise," *Newsweek*, January 14, 2020, https://www.newsweek.com/what-so-called-deaths-despair-experts-say-rise-1481975; Atul Gawande, "Why Americans Are Dying from Despair," *The New Yorker*, March 16, 2020, https://www.newyorker.com/magazine/2020/03/23/why-americans-are-dying-from-despair; Jamie Ducharme, "More Millennials Are Dying 'Deaths of Despair,' as Overdose and Suicide Rates Climb," *TIME*, June 13, 2019, https://time.com/5606411/millennials-deaths-of-despair/.

27. Becky Bach, "Suicide and Other 'Deaths of Despair' Are Vexing, but Preventable, Speakers Say," Scope, Stanford Medicine, March 1, 2019, https://scopeblog.stanford.edu/2019/03/01/suicide-and-other-deaths-of-despair-are-vexing-but-preventable-speakers-say/.

28. Alec Coppen and Christina Bolander-Gouaille, "Treatment of Depression: Time to Consider Folic Acid and Vitamin B12," *Journal of Psychopharmacology* 19, no. 1 (2005): 59–65, https://doi.org/10.1177/0269881105048899; Nicolas Singewald *et al.*,

"Magnesium-Deficient Diet Alters Depression- and Anxiety-Related Behavior in Mice—Influence of Desipramine and *Hypericum perforatum* Extract," *Neuropharmacology* 47, no. 8 (December 2004): 1189–97, https://doi.org/10.1016/j.neuropharm.2004.08.010.

29. A. Sánchez-Villegas *et al.*, "Mediterranean Diet and Depression," *Public Health Nutrition* 9, no. 8A (2006): 1104–9, https://doi.org/10.1017/S1368980007668578.

30. Monique Tello, "Diet and Depression," Harvard Health Blog, February 22, 2018, https://www.health.harvard.edu/blog/diet-and-depression-2018022213309; Shae E. Quirk *et al.*, "The Association Between Diet Quality, Dietary Patterns and Depression in Adults: A Systematic Review," *BMC Psychiatry* 13 (2013): 175, https://doi.org/10.1186/1471-244X-13-175.

31. David Railton, "Natural Remedies for Treating Bipolar Disorder," Medical News Today, October 10, 2018, https://www.medicalnewstoday.com/articles/314435.

32. University of Oxford, "Many Mental Illnesses Reduce Life Expectancy More Than Heavy Smoking," ScienceDaily, May 23, 2014, https://www.sciencedaily.com/releases/2014/05/140523082934.htm.

33. Brenda Jensen, Charles T. Nguyen, and Gerald A. Maguire, "Bipolar Disorder: Increasing the Effectiveness and Decreasing the Side Effects of Treatment," *Psychiatric Times* 2, no. 24 (February 11, 2007), https://www.psychrictimes.com/view/bipolar-disorder-increasing-effectiveness-and-decreasing-side-effects-treatment; Carolyn L. Turvey *et al.*, "Long-Term Prognosis of Bipolar I Disorder," *Acta Psychiatrica Scandinavica* 99, no. 2 (February 1999): 110–19, https://doi.org/10.1111/j.1600-0447.1999.tb07208.x.

34. L. V. Kessing, "Does the Risk of Developing Dementia Increase with the Number of Episodes in Patients with Depressive Disorder and in Patients with Bipolar Disorder?," *Journal of Neurology, Neurosurgery & Psychiatry* 75, no. 12 (2004): 1662–66, https://doi.org/10.1136/jnnp.2003.031773.

35. Michael J. Gitlin, "Antidepressants in Bipolar Depression: An Enduring Controversy," *International Journal of Bipolar Disorders* 6 (2018): article 25, https://dx.doi.org/10.1186/s40345-018-0133-9.

36. Elisa F. Cascade *et al.*, "Antidepressants in Bipolar Disorder," *Psychiatry (Edgmont)* 4, no. 3 (March 2007): 56–58, https://www.ncbi.nlm.nih.gov/pmc/articles/PMC2922360/; Mitsuhiro Tada *et al.*, "Antidepressant Dose and Treatment Response in Bipolar Depression: Reanalysis of the Systematic Treatment Enhancement Program for Bipolar Disorder (STEP-BD) Data," *Journal of Psychiatric Research* 68 (September 2015): 151–56, https://doi.org/10.1016/j.jpsychires.2015.06.015.

37. Joseph F. Goldberg, "Antidepressants in Bipolar Disorder: 7 Myths and Realities," *Current Psychiatry* 9, no. 5 (May 2010): 41–49, https://www.mdedge.com/psychiatry/article/63888/bipolar-disorder/antidepressants-bipolar-disorder-7-myths-and-realities.

38. J. A. Stoukides and C. A. Stoukides, "Extrapyramidal Symptoms upon Discontinuation of Fluoxetine," *American Journal of Psychiatry* 148, no. 9 (September 1991): 1263, https://doi.org/10.1176/ajp.148.9.1263a; Peter C. Groot and Jim van Os, "How User Knowledge of Psychotropic Drug Withdrawal Resulted in the Development of Person-Specific Tapering Medication," *Therapeutic Advances in Psychopharmacology* 10 (January 2020), https://doi.org/10.1177/2045125320932452.

39. A. F. Schatzberg *et al.*, "Serotonin Reuptake Inhibitor Discontinuation Syndrome: A Hypothetical Definition. Discontinuation Consensus Panel," *Journal of Clinical Psychiatry* 58, no. S7 (1997): 5–10; Peter Haddad, Michel Lejoyeux, and Allan Young, "Antidepressant Discontinuation Reactions: Are Preventable and Simple to Treat," *BMJ* 316, no. 7138 (April 1998): 1105–6, https://doi.org/10.1136/bmj.316.7138.1105; Peter

Haddad, "The SSRI Discontinuation Syndrome," *Journal of Psychopharmacology* 12, no. 3 (1998): 305–13, https://doi.org/10.1177%2F026988119801200311.

40. William Schultz and Noel Hunter, "Depression, Chemical Imbalances, and Feminism," *Journal of Feminist Family Therapy* 28, no. 4 (2016): 159–73, https://doi.org/10.1080/0 8952833.2016.1235523; Taneasha White, "Family-Centered Programs May Help Protect Black Youth from Effects of Racism," Verywell Mind, April 13, 2021, https://www .verywellmind.com/family-centered-programs-protect-black-youth-5120307; Charlotte Blease, "The Duty to Be Well-Informed: The Case of Depression," *Journal of Medical Ethics* 40 (March 2014): 225–29, https://jme.bmj.com/content/40/4/225; Jeffrey R. Lacasse and Jonathan Leo, "Serotonin and Depression: A Disconnect between the Advertisements and the Scientific Literature," *PLoS Medicine* 2, no. 12 (2005): e392, https://doi.org/10.1371/journal.pmed.0020392; Hal Arkowitz and Scott O. Lilienfeld, "Is Depression Just Bad Chemistry?," *Scientific American*, March 1, 2014, https://www .scientificamerican.com/article/is-depression-just-bad-chemistry/.

41. J. J. Schildkraut, "The Catecholamine Hypothesis of Affective Disorders: A Review of Supporting Evidence," *American Journal of Psychiatry* 122, no. 5 (November 1965): 509–22, https://doi.org/10.1176/ajp.122.5.509.

42. Irving Kirsch and Guy Sapirstein, "Listening to Prozac but Hearing Placebo: A Meta-Analysis of Antidepressant Medication," *Prevention & Treatment* 1, no. 2 (1998): article 2a, https://doi.org/10.1037/1522-3736.1.1.12a.

43. Irving Kirsch, "Antidepressants and the Placebo Effect," *Zeitschrift Fur Psychologie* 222, no. 3 (2014): 128–34, https://doi.org/10.1027/2151-2604/a000176.

44. Steve Stewart-Williams and John Podd, "The Placebo Effect: Dissolving the Expectancy Versus Conditioning Debate," *Psychological Bulletin* 130, no.2 (2004): 324–40. https://doi.org/10.1037/0033-2909.130.2.324.

45. Marcia Angell, "The Epidemic of Mental Illness: Why?" *New York Review of Books*, June 23, 2011, https://www.nybooks.com/articles/2011/06/23/epidemic-mental-illness -why/.

46. Florida State University, "Media Perpetuates Unsubstantiated Chemical Imbalance Theory of Depression, Study Shows," ScienceDaily, March 3, 2008, https://www.science daily.com/releases/2008/03/080303164507.htm; Jonathan Leo and Jeffrey R. Lacasse, "The Media and the Chemical Imbalance Theory of Depression," *Society* 45 (2008): 35–45, https://doi.org/10.1007/s12115-007-9047-3.

47. Harrington, *Mind Fixers*, 201; Thomas Fleming, "What's Happening in Psychiatry? Or, Where Are All the Analysts Hiding?," *Cosmopolitan*, March 1970, 164–67, 182–83; Richard M. Restak, "Researchers Seek to Aid the Treatment of Emotional Illness," *New York Times*, December 12, 1976, https://www.nytimes.com/1976/12/12 /archives/researchers-seek-to-aid-the-treatment-of-emotional-illness-some.html; John Noble Wilford, "Pauling Links Mental Ills to Chemical Imbalance; Scientist Says Heredity or Diet Could Cause the Condition Suggests Restoring Balance in the Brain Is Best Therapy," *New York Times*, April 20, 1968, https://www.nytimes.com/1968/04 /20/archives/pauling-links-mental-ills-to-chemical-imbalance-scientist-says.html.

48. Jacquelyn Cafasso, "Chemical Imbalance in the Brain: What You Should Know" (Healthline, February 9, 2021), https://www.healthline.com/health/chemical-imbalance -in-the-brain.

49. Ronald W. Pies, "Debunking the Two Chemical Imbalance Myths, Again," *Psychiatric Times* 36, no. 8 (August 2, 2019), https://www.psychiatrictimes.com/debunking-two -chemical-imbalance-myths-again/page/0/3.

50. Leo and Lacasse, "The Media and the Chemical Imbalance Theory of Depression";

Ronald Pies, "Nuances, Narratives, and the 'Chemical Imbalance' Debate," *Psychiatric Times* 31, no. 4 (April 11, 2014), https://www.psychiatrictimes.com/view/nuances-narratives-and-chemical-imbalance-debate.

51. Joshua J. Kemp, James J. Lickel, and Brett J. Deacon, "Effects of a Chemical Imbalance Causal Explanation of Individuals' Perceptions of Their Depressive Symptoms," Behaviour Research and Therapy 56 (May 2014): 47–52, https://doi.org/10.1016/j.brat.2014.02.009.

52. Andreasen, *Broken Brain*, 29.

53. Fred Baughman, "There Is No Such Thing as a Psychiatric Disorder/Disease/Chemical Imbalance," *PLoS Medicine* 3, no. 7 (July 2006): e318, https://dx.doi.org/10.1371/journal.pmed.0030318; Woo-Kyoung Ahn, Caroline C. Proctor, and Elizabeth H. Flanagan, "Mental Health Clinicians' Beliefs About the Biological, Psychological, and Environmental Bases of Mental Disorders," *Cognitive Science* 33, no. 2 (March/April 2009): 147–82, https://dx.doi.org/10.1111/j.1551-6709.2009.01008.x.

54. J. H. Chauvier, *A Treatise on Punctuation* (1849), trans. J. B. Huntington (Whitefish, MT: Kessinger Publishing, 2010).

11. On Suicidal Ideation

1. Al and Cake, "An Interview with . . . Kurt Cobain," *Flipside*, May/June 1992, http://www.nirvanaclub.com/info/articles/05.00.92-flipside.html.

2. Stefan G. Hofmann *et al.*, "The Efficacy of Cognitive Behavioral Therapy: A Review of Meta-Analyses," *Cognitive Therapy and Research* 36 (2012): 427–40, https://doi.org/10.1007/s10608-012-9476-1; Andrew C. Butler *et al.*, "The Empirical Status of Cognitive-Behavioral Therapy: A Review of Meta-Analysis," *Clinical Psychology Review* 26, no. 1 (January 2006): 17–31, https://doi.org/10.1016/j.cpr.2005.07.003.

3. David Burns, *When Panic Attacks: The New, Drug-Free Anxiety Therapy That Can Change Your Life* (New York: Random House, 2006), Kindle.

4. R. Haussmann *et al.*, "Treatment of Lithium Intoxication: Facing the Need for Evidence," *International Journal of Bipolar Disorders* 3, no. 1 (2015): article 23, https://doi.org/10.1186/s40345-015-0040-2.

5. David A. Cousins *et al.*, "Lithium: Past, Present, and Future," *The Lancet Psychiatry* 7, no. 3 (March 2020): 222–24, https://doi.org/10.1016/S2215-0366(19)30365-7.

6. Alan D. Strobusch and James W. Jefferson, "The Checkered History of Lithium in Medicine," *Pharmacy in History* 22, no. 2 (1980): 72–76, https://www.jstor.org/stable/41109216?seq=1.

7. Lawrence W. Hanlon *et al.*, "Lithium Chloride as a Substitute for Sodium Chloride in the Diet: Observations on Its Toxicity," *JAMA* 139, no. 11 (1949): 688–92, https://doi.org/10.1001/jama.1949.02900280004002.

8. Fred Kleinsinger, "Working with the Noncompliant Patient," *The Permanente Journal* 14, no. 1 (Spring 2010): 54–60, https://doi.org/10.7812/tpp/09-064.

9. Lars Osterberg and Terrence Blaschke, "Adherence to Medication," *The New England Journal of Medicine* 353, no. 5 (2005): 487–97, https://doi.org/10.1056/NEJMra050100.

10. Katalin Szanto *et al.*, "Suicide in Elderly Depressed Patients: Is Active vs. Passive Suicidal Ideation a Clinically Valid Distinction?," *The American Journal of Geriatric Psychiatry* 4, no. 3 (Summer 1996): 197–207, https://doi.org/10.1097/00019442-199622430-00003.

11. Enrique Baca-Garcia *et al.*, "Estimating Risk for Suicide Attempt: Are We Asking the Right Questions?: Passive Suicidal Ideation as a Marker for Suicidal Behavior,"

Journal of Affective Disorders 134, no. 1–3 (November 2011): 327–32, https://dx.doi .org/10.1016%2Fj.jad.2011.06.026.

12. Aaron T. Beck, Maria Kovacs, and Arlene Weissman, "Assessment of Suicidal Intention: The Scale for Suicide Ideation," *Journal of Consulting and Clinical Psychology* 47, no. 2 (May 1979): 343–52, http://dx.doi.org/10.1037/0022-006X.47.2.343.

13. Peter Tarr, "Homelessness and Mental Illness: A Challenge to Our Society," Brain and Behavior Research Foundation, November 19, 2018, https://www.bbrfoundation .org/blog/homelessness-and-mental-illness-challenge-our-society; "HUD Exchange, 2015 AHAR: Part 1—PIT Estimates of Homelessness in the U.S.," US Department of Housing and Urban Development, November 2015, https://www.hudexchange .info/resource/4832/2015-ahar-part-1-pit-estimates-of-homelessness/.

14. Sourav Khanra and Basudeb Das, "Off-Label Psychotropics Use: Isn't It Now an Inevitable and a 'Norm' in Psychiatry?," *Indian Journal of Psychological Medicine* 40, no. 4 (July 2018): 390–91, https://dx.doi.org/10.4103%2FIJPSYM.IJPSYM_563_17; Christopher M. Wittich, Christopher M. Burkle, and William L. Lanier, "Ten Common Questions (and Their Answers) about Off-label Drug Use," *Mayo Clinic Proceedings* 87, no. 10 (October 2012): 982–90, https://dx.doi.org/10.1016%2Fj.mayocp.2012.04 .017; Darhan Kharadi *et al.*, "Off-Label Drug Use in Psychiatry Outpatient Department: A Prospective Study at a Tertiary Care Teaching Hospital," *Journal of Basic and Clinical Pharmacy* 6, no. 2 (May 2015): 45–49, https://dx.doi.org/10.4103%2F 0976-0105.152090.

15. Ronald Pies, "Should Psychiatrists Use Atypical Antipsychotics to Treat Nonpsychotic Anxiety?," *Psychiatry (Edgmont)* 6, no. 6 (June 2009): 29–37, https://www.ncbi .nlm.nih.gov/pmc/articles/PMC2720845/; Artie Berns, "Dementia and Antipsychotics: A Prescription for Problems," *Journal of Legal Medicine* 33, no. 4 (2012): 553–69, https://doi.org/10.1080/01947648.2012.739067; M. El Gewely *et al.*, "The Off-Label Use of Antipsychotics for Insomnia Disorder: A Major Public Health Concern," *Sleep Medicine* 64, no. 1 (December 2019): S103, https://doi.org/10.1016/j.sleep.2019.11.282.

16. "Understanding Unapproved Use of Approved Drugs 'Off Label,'" US Food and Drug Administration, February 5, 2018, https://www.fda.gov/patients/learn-about -expanded-access-and-other-treatment-options/understanding-unapproved-use -approved-drugs-label.

17. Louise Carton et al., "Off-Label Prescribing of Antipsychotics in Adults, Children and Elderly Individuals: A Systematic Review of Recent Prescription Trends," *Current Pharmaceutical Design* 21, no. 23 (2015): 3280–97, https://doi.org/10.2174/138161282 1666150619092903.

18. Cathy L. Melvin *et al.*, "Marketing Off-Label Uses: Shady Practices within a Gray Market," *Psychiatric Times* 26, no. 8 (August 7, 2009), https://www.psychiatrictimes .com/view/marketing-label-uses-shady-practices-within-gray-market; Stephanie Saul, "Experts Conclude Pfizer Manipulated Studies," *New York Times*, October 8, 2008, https://www.nytimes.com/2008/10/08/health/research/08drug.html.

19. Wittich, Burkle, and Lanier, "Ten Common Questions."

20. Gardiner Harris, "Drug Makers Are Advocacy Group's Biggest Donors," *New York Times*, October 21, 2009, https://www.nytimes.com/2009/10/22/health/22nami.html; Katherine Hobson, "Mental Health Group's State Chapters Get Millions from Pharma," *Wall Street Journal*, April 28, 2010, https://www.wsj.com/articles/BL-HEB-33035.

21. Martha Rosenberg, "Pharma Funding Advocacy Groups," Center for Health Journalism, October 15, 2014, https://centerforhealthjournalism.org/2014/10/15/discredited -patient-group-fights-mental-illness.

22. College of Psychiatric and Neurologic Pharmacists, "Off-Label Usage of Medications," National Alliance on Mental Health Illness, March 2019, https://www.nami.org/Learn-More/Treatment/Mental-Health-Medications/Off-Label-Usage-of-Medications; "Medications for Mood Disorders," Depression and Bipolar Support Alliance, https://www.dbsalliance.org/wellness/treatment-options/medications/; Andrew Adesman, "What to Do When You Can't Get the ADHD Medication You Want," Children and Adults with Attention-Deficit/Hyperactivity Disorder (CHADD), June 2018, https://chadd.org/attention-article/what-to-do-when-you-cant-get-the-adhd-medication-you-want/; Melvin *et al.*, "Marketing Off-Label Uses."

23. Tamara Pringsheim *et al.*, "The Assessment and Treatment of Antipsychotic-Induced Akathisia," *The Canadian Journal of Psychiatry* 63, no. 11 (2018): 719–29, https://doi.org/10.1177/0706743718760288.

24. Haitham Salem *et al.*, "Revisiting Antipsychotic-Induced Akathisia: Current Issues and Prospective Challenges," *Current Neuropharmacology* 15, no. 5 (July 2017): 789–98, https://dx.doi.org/10.2174%2F1570159X14666161208153644.

25. "Haldol Tablet," WebMD, https://www.webmd.com/drugs/2/drug-5419/haldol-oral/details; sinaiem, "Can't Sedate Me! I'm Allergic to Haldol," Mount Sinai Emergency Medicine, November 12, 2015, https://sinaiem.org/cant-sedate-me-im-allergic-to-haldol/.

26. Rosie Harding and Elizabeth Peel, "'Zombie Drugs,'" OUPblog, November 28, 2012, https://blog.oup.com/2012/11/zombie-drugsantipsychotics-dementia/.

27. Cecelia Watson, *Semicolon: The Past, Present, and Future of a Misunderstood Mark* (New York: Ecco, 2019), 16, Kindle.

28. Watson, *Semicolon* 49.

29. Project *Semicolon*, 2019, https://projectsemicolon.com.

12. "Sick"

1. David Crystal, *Making a Point: The Persnickety Story of English Punctuation* (New York: St. Martin's Publishing Group, 2015), Kindle.

2. Ruth Finnegan, *Why Do We Quote?: The Culture and History of Quotation* (Cambridge, UK: Open Book Publishers, 2011), 86–87; Keith Houston, *Shady Characters: The Secret Life of Punctuation, Symbols, and Other Typographical Marks* (New York: W. W. Norton, 2013).

3. Bernard Fischer, "A Review of American Psychiatry through Its Diagnoses: The History and Development of the Diagnostic and Statistical Manual of Mental Disorders," *The Journal of Nervous and Mental Disease* 200, no. 12 (December 2012): 1022–30, https://doi.org/10.1097/NMD.0b013e318275cf19.

4. Blashfield *et al.*, "The Cycle of Classification."

5. American Psychiatric Association, *The People Behind DSM-5*, Fact Sheet, 2013, https://www.psychiatry.org/psychiatrists/practice/dsm/educational-resources/dsm-5-fact-sheets.

6. Charles B. Nemeroff *et al.*, "DSM-5: A Collection of Psychiatrist Views on the Changes, Controversies, and Future Directions," *BMC Medicine* 1, (2013): article 202, https://doi.org/10.1186/1741-7015-11-202; E. M. Shackle, "Psychiatric Diagnosis as an Ethical Problem," *Journal of Medical Ethics* 11, no. 3 (1985): 132–34, https://doi.org/10.1136/jme.11.3.132.

7. Ronald Pies, "Should DSM-V Designate 'Internet Addiction' a Mental Disorder?" *Psychiatry (Edgmont)* 6, no. 2 (February 2009): 31–37.

8. Kendler, Muñoz, and Murphy, "The Development of the Feighner Criteria."

9. Hannah S. Decker, "How Kraepelinian Was Kraepelin? How Kraepelinian Are the Neo-Kraepelinians?—from Emil Kraepelin to DSM-III," *History of Psychiatry* 18, no. 3 (2007): 337–60, https://doi.org/10.1177/0957154X07078976.

10. Relying on Blashfield's number—*DSM-III* had 228.

11. Kendler, Muñoz, and Murphy, "The Development of the Feighner Criteria."

12. Hannah Decker, *The Making of DSM-III®: A Diagnostic Manual's Conquest of American Psychiatry* (Cary: Oxford University Press, 2013), 139, ProQuest Ebook Central.

13. Horwitz, *DSM*, 57.

14. Stuart A. Kirk and Herb Kutchins, *The Selling of DSM: The Rhetoric of Science in Psychiatry* (New York: Routledge, 1992), 185.

15. Allen J. Frances, Thomas A. Widiger, and Harold Alan Pincus, "The Development of DSM-IV," *Archives of General Psychiatry* 46, no. 4 (1989): 373–75, https://doi.org/10.1001/archpsyc.1989.01810040079012.

16. Meagenda, "APA News Release: 09 March 10: APA Modifies DSM Naming Convention to Reflect Publication Changes," Dx Revision Watch, March 9, 2010, https://dxrevisionwatch.com/2010/03/09/apa-news-release-09-march-10-apa-modifies-dsm-naming-convention-to-reflect-publication-changes/.

17. Frances, *Saving Normal*, 173.

18. Paula J. Caplan, *They Say You're Crazy: How the World's Most Powerful Psychiatrists Decide Who's Normal* (Reading, PA: Addison-Wesley, 1995), 186.

19. Caplan, *They Say You're Crazy*, 195.

20. Peter Tyrer, "A Comparison of DSM and ICD Classifications of Mental Disorder," *Advances in Psychiatric Treatment* 20, no. 4 (2014), 280–85, https://doi.org/10.1192/apt.bp.113.011296.

21. Decker, *The Making of DSM-III*, 139.

22. S. Nassir Ghaemi, "Why DSM-III, IV, and 5 Are Unscientific," Psychiatric Times, October 14, 2013, https://www.psychiatrictimes.com/view/why-dsm-iii-iv-and-5-are-unscientific.

23. Todd Dufresne, "Psychoanalysis Is Dead . . . So How Does That Make You Feel?," *Los Angeles Times*, February 18, 2004, https://www.latimes.com/archives/la-xpm-2004-feb-18-oe-dufresne18-story.html.

24. Ernst Falzeder, "The Story of an Ambivalent Relationship: Sigmund Freud and Eugen Bleuler," *Journal of Analytical Psychology* 52, no. 3 (June 2007): 343–68, https://doi.org/10.1111/j.1468-5922.2007.00666.x.

25. Susan V. Eisen, Barbara Dickey, and Lloyd I. Sederer, "A Self-Report Symptom and Problem Rating Scale to Increase Inpatients' Involvement in Treatment," *Psychiatric Services* 51, no. 3 (March 2000): 349–53, https://doi.org/10.1176/appi.ps.51.3.349; Sara Evans-Lacko *et al.*, "Psychometric Validation of the Self-Identification of Having a Mental Illness (SELF-I) Scale and the Relationship with Stigma and Help-Seeking among Young People," *Social Psychiatry and Psychiatric Epidemiology* 54, no. 1 (January 2019): 59–67, https://doi.org/10.1007/s00127-018-1602-2.

26. Georg Schomerus *et al.*, "Validity and Psychometric Properties of the Self-Identification as Having a Mental Illness Scale (SELF-I) among Currently Untreated Persons with Mental Health Problems," *Psychiatry Research* 273 (March 2019): 303–8, https://doi.org/10.1016/j.psychres.2019.01.054.

13. On Solitude (and Isolation and Loneliness [and Brackets])

1. Frances, *Saving Normal*, 221.
2. Horwitz and Wakefield, *Loss of Sadness*, 19.
3. Greenberg, *Book of Woe*, 346.
4. Florence Hazrat, "Pause and Effect," *History Today* 70, no. 2 (February 2020), https://www.historytoday.com/history-matters/pause-and-effect.

14. On Stigma (and Disclosure)

1. Tahirah Abdullah and Tamara L. Brown, "Mental Illness Stigma and Ethnocultural Beliefs, Values, and Norms: An Investigative Review," *Clinical Psychology Review* 31, no. 6 (August 2011): 934–48, https://doi.org/10.1016/j.cpr.2011.05.003.
2. "Suicide Rates Rising across the U.S.: Comprehensive Prevention Goes Beyond a Focus on Mental Health Concerns," Centers for Disease Control and Prevention, June 7, 2018, https://www.cdc.gov/media/releases/2018/p0607-suicide-prevention.html.
3. María A. Oquendo and Enrique Baca-Garcia, "Suicidal Behavior Disorder as a Diagnostic Entity in the DSM-5 Classification System: Advantages Outweigh Limitations," *World Psychiatry* 13, no. 2 (June 2014): 128–30, https://dx.doi.org/10.1002%2Fwps.20116; Oquendo *et al.*, "Issues for DSM-V."
4. E. A. Gjelten, "Illinois Misdemeanor Crimes by Class and Sentences," Criminal Defense Lawyer, https://www.criminaldefenselawyer.com/resources/illinois-misdemeanor-crimes-class-and-sentences.htm.
5. James Warren, "Socratic Suicide," *The Journal of Hellenic Studies* 121 (2001): 91–106, https://doi.org/10.2307/631830.
6. Miriam Griffin, "Philosophy, Cato, and Roman Suicide: II," *Greece and Rome* 33, no. 2 (1986): 192–202, https://doi.org/10.1017/S0017383500030357.
7. L. R. Kirkland, "To End Itself by Death: Suicide in Shakespeare's Tragedies," *Southern Medical Journal* 92, no. 7 (July 1999): 660–66, https://pubmed.ncbi.nlm.nih.gov/10414473/.
8. Eugenio Lecaldano, "Hume on Suicide," in *The Oxford Handbook of Hume*, ed. Paul Russell (New York: Oxford University Press, 2016), 660–72, https://doi.org/10.1093/oxfordhb/9780199742844.013.14.
9. Terri L. Snyder, *The Power to Die: Slavery and Suicide in British North America* (Chicago: University of Chicago Press, 2015).
10. Émile Durkheim, *Suicide: A Study in Sociology* (London: Routledge, 1951), https://doi.org/10.4324/9780203994320.
11. Daniel R. Mistich, review of *Suicide: Foucault, History and Truth, by Ian Marsh, Foucault Studies* 16 (September 2013): 208–11, https://doi.org/10.22439/fs.v0i16.4133.
12. Benedict Carey and Robert Gebeloff, "Many People Taking Antidepressants Discover They Cannot Quit," *New York Times*, April 7, 2018, https://www.nytimes.com/2018/04/07/health/antidepressants-withdrawal-prozac-cymbalta.html.
13. Rachel Aviv, "The Challenge of Going Off Psychiatric Drugs," *The New Yorker*, April 8, 2019, https://www.newyorker.com/magazine/2019/04/08/the-challenge-of-going-off-psychiatric-drugs.
14. "The Medication Debate: Time to Change the Record," *The Lancet Psychiatry* 5, no. 10 (October 2018): 769, https://doi.org/10.1016/S2215-0366(18)30359-6; Mark Moran, "Experts Debate Effects of Antidepressant Warning," *Psychiatric News* 49, no. 23 (December 2014), https://doi.org/10.1176/appi.pn.2014.12a3; Intelligence Squared,

"Psychiatrists and the Pharma Industry Are to Blame for the Current 'Epidemic' of Mental Disorders," YouTube video, May 11, 2015, 1:32:05, https://www.youtube.com /watch?v=GlFbuqunb1I; "Are Psychiatric Drugs Doing More Harm Than Good? Kings College London Maudsley Annotated Debate," Ragged University, May 2015, https:// www.raggeduniversity.co.uk/2016/11/08/are-psychiatric-drugs-doing-more-harm-than -good-kings-college-london-maudsley-annotated-debate/; "Current Controversies in Psychiatry," BioMedCentral, accessed August 2020, https://www.biomedcentral .com/collections/CCP; Stephen Ginn, "Prozac Notion," *The Lancet* 388, no. 10062 (December 2016): 2860, https://doi.org/10.1016/S0140-6736(16)32471-0; Open Excel-lence, "2015 Yale Symposium—David Healy, MD, FRCPsych," YouTube video, May 8, 2015, 43:31, https://www.youtube.com/watch?v=23lH5xTPYpM&feature=youtu.be; Cardiff University Psychology, "David Healy—Hearts and Minds: Psychotropic Drugs and Violence," YouTube video, May 29, 2013, 56:35, https://www.youtube.com/watch ?v=CCta8I0pKqM&feature=youtu.be.

15. Swapnil Gupta and John Daniel Cahill, "A Prescription for 'Deprescribing' in Psychi-atry," *Psychiatric Services* 67, no. 8 (August 2016): 904–7, https://doi.org/10.1176/appi .ps.201500359.

16. Tim Hains, "Dr. Peter Breggin: Psychiatrists Have Gone 'Mad' for Prescribing Medica-tion," Real Clear Politics, March 17, 2019, https://www.realclearpolitics.com/video/2019 /03/17/dr_peter_breggin_psychiatrists_have_gone_mad_for_prescribing_medication.html.

17. Robert Whitaker, "Psychiatry Defends Its Antipsychotics: A Case Study of Institutional Corruption," Mad in America, May 21, 2017, https://www.madinamerica.com/2017/05 /psychiatry-defends-its-antipsychotics-case-study-of-institutional-corruption/; Miriam Larsen Barr, "Responding to Claims that the Benefits of Antipsychotics Outweigh the Risks," Mad in America, May 6, 2017, https://www.madinamerica.com/2017/05/ responding-to-claims-that-the-benefits-of-antipsychotics-outweigh-the-risks/; Joanna Moncrieff, "Inconvenient Truths about Antipsychotics: A Response to Goff et al," Mad in America May 7, 2017, https://www.madinamerica.com/2017/05/inconvenient -truths-about-antipsychotics-a-response-to-goff-et-al/; Donald C. Goff et al., "The Long-Term Effects of Antipsychotic Medication on Clinical Course in Schizophre-nia," *American Journal of Psychiatry* 174, no. 9 (September 2017): 840–49, https://doi .org/10.1176/appi.ajp.2017.16091016; Peter Gøtzsche, "Myths about Antidepressants & Antipsychotics," Davidhealy.org, January 21, 2014. https://davidhealy.org/psychiatry -gone-astray/.

18. John Lennard, *The Poetry Handbook: A Guide to Reading Poetry for Pleasure and Practical Criticism*, 2nd ed. (Oxford: Oxford University Press, 2005), 123.

Epilogue

1. George M. Beard, "The Psychology of Spiritism," *The North American Review* 129, no. 272 (July 1879): 65–80, www.jstor.org/stable/25100777.

2. Association for Psychological Science, "The Power of Suggestion: What We Expect Influences Our Behavior, for Better or Worse," ScienceDaily, June 6, 2012, https://www .sciencedaily.com/releases/2012/06/120606142818.htm.

3. Edward H. Hagen, "Evolutionary Theories of Depression: A Critical Review," *The Canadian Journal of Psychiatry* 56, no. 12 (December 2011): 716–26, https://doi.org /10.1177/070674371105601203.

4. Randolph M. Nesse, *Good Reasons for Bad Feelings: Insights from the Frontier of Evolutionary Psychiatry* (New York: Dutton, 2019), Kindle.

5. Henri-Jean Aubin, Ivan Berlin, and Charles Kornreich, "The Evolutionary Puzzle of Suicide," *International Journal of Environmental Research and Public Health* 10, no. 12 (December 2013): 6873–86, https://dx.doi.org/10.3390/ijerph10126873.

6. J. John Mann, Victoria Arango, and Mark D. Underwood, "Serotonin and Suicidal Behavior," *Annals of the New York Academy of Sciences* 600, no. 1 (October 1990): 476–84, https://doi.org/10.1111/j.1749-6632.1990.tb16903.x; Erik Ryding, Mats Lindström, and Lil Träskman-Bendz, "The Role of Dopamine and Serotonin in Suicidal Behavior and Aggression," *Progress in Brain Research* 172 (2008): 307–15, https://doi.org/10.1016/S0079-6123(08)00915-1; Catherine Offord, "What Neurobiology Can Tell Us about Suicide," The Scientist, January 13, 2020, https://www.the-scientist.com/features/what-neurobiology-can-tell-us-about-suicide-66922; J. John Mann *et al.*, "Candidate Endophenotypes for Genetic Studies of Suicidal Behavior," *Biological Psychiatry* 65, no. 7 (April 2009): 556–63, https://dx.doi.org/10.1016%2Fj.biopsych.2008.11.021; Dan Rujescu *et al.*, "Genetic Variations in Tryptophan Hydroxylase in Suicidal Behavior: Analysis and Meta-Analysis," *Biological Psychiatry* 54, no. 4 (August 2003): 465–73, https://doi.org/10.1016/S0006-3223(02)01748-1; Vikas Menon and Shivanand Kattimani, "Suicide and Serotonin: Making Sense of Evidence," *Indian Journal of Psychological Medicine* 37, no. 3 (July 2015): 377–78, https://dx.doi.org/10.4103%2F0253-7176.162910; Clement C. Zai *et al.*, "Genetic Factors and Suicidal Behavior," chap. 11 in *The Neurobiological Basis of Suicide*, ed. Yogesh Dwivedi (Boca Raton, FL: Taylor and Francis, 2012).

7. Lisa Cosgrove and Sheldon Krimsky, "A Comparison of *DSM-IV* and *DSM-5* Panel Members' Financial Associations with Industry: A Pernicious Problem Persists," *PLoS Medicine* 9, no. 3 (2012): e1001190, https://doi.org/10.1371/journal.pmed.1001190.

8. Taeho Greg Rhee and Samuel T Wilkinson, "Exploring the Psychiatrist-Industry Financial Relationship: Insight from the Open Payment Data of Centers for Medicare and Medicaid Services," *Administration and Policy in Mental Health* 47, no. 4 (2020): 526–30, https://doi.org/10.1007/s10488-020-01009-2.

9. Gardiner Harris, "Research Center Tied to Drug Company," *New York Times*, November 24, 2008, https://www.nytimes.com/2008/11/25/health/25psych.html?ref=joseph_biederman.

10. Gardiner Harris, "Top Psychiatrist Didn't Report Drug Makers' Pay," *New York Times*, October 3, 2008, https://www.nytimes.com/2008/10/04/health/policy/04drug.html; Gardiner Harris, "Drug Maker Told Studies Would Aid It, Papers Say," *New York Times*, March 19, 2009, https://www.nytimes.com/2009/03/20/us/20psych.html; Katie Thomas, "J.&J. to Pay $2.2 Billion in Risperdal Settlement," *New York Times*, November 4, 2013, https://www.nytimes.com/2013/11/05/business/johnson-johnson-to-settle-risperdal-improper-marketing-case.html.

11. Gardiner Harris, "3 Researchers at Harvard Are Named in Subpoena," *New York Times*, March 27, 2009, https://www.nytimes.com/2009/03/28/health/policy/28subpoena.html.

12. Liz Kowalczyk, "Harvard Doctors Punished Over Pay," Boston.com, July 2, 2011, http://archive.boston.com/news/local/massachusetts/articles/2011/07/02/three_harvard_psychiatrists_are_sanctioned_over_consulting_fees/; Xi Yu, "Three Professors Face Sanctions Following Harvard Medical School Inquiry," *The Harvard Crimson*, July 2, 2011, https://www.thecrimson.com/article/2011/7/2/school-medical-harvard-investigation/.

13. Koerner, "First, You Market the Disease…"

14. Ken Silverstein, "Prozac.org," *Mother Jones*, November/December 1999, https://www .motherjones.com/politics/1999/11/prozacorg/.

15. D. A. Regier *et al.*, "The NIMH Depression Awareness, Recognition, and Treatment Program: Structure, Aims, and Scientific Basis," *American Journal of Psychiatry* 145, no. 11 (November 1988): 1351–57, https://doi.org/10.1176/ajp.145.11.1351; Whitaker, *Anatomy of an Epidemic*, 279.

16. John Sadler, "Considering the Economy of DSM Alternatives," in *Making the DSM-5: Concepts and Controversies*, ed. J. Paris and J. Phillips (New York: Springer Nature, 2013), 21–38, https://psycnet.apa.org/doi/10.1007/978-1-4614-6504-1_2.

17. Jerome C. Wakefield, "DSM-5, Psychiatric Epidemiology and the False Positives Problem," *Epidemiology and Psychiatric Sciences* 24, no. 3 (2015): 188–96, https://doi .org/10.1017/S2045796015000116.

18. Robert Kendell, "Distinguishing Between the Validity and Utility of Psychiatric Diagnoses," *American Journal of Psychiatry* 160, no. 1 (January 2003): 4–12, https://doi .org/10.1176/appi.ajp.160.1.4.

19. Assen Jablensky, "Psychiatric Classifications: Validity and Utility," *World Psychiatry (Edgmont)* 15, no. 1 (February 2016): 26–31, https://dx.doi.org/10.1002/wps.20284.

20. Michael Marshall, "The Hidden Links between Mental Disorders," *Nature* 581, no. 7806 (2020): 19–21, https://doi.org/10.1038/d41586-020-00922-8; Jonathan Leo and Jeffrey R. Lacasse, "The Media and the Chemical Imbalance Theory of Depression," *Society* 45 (2008): 35–45, https://doi.org/10.1007/s12115-007-9047-3.

21. A. Scull, "American Psychiatry in the New Millennium: A Critical Appraisal," *Psychological Medicine* 51, no. 16 (2021): 2762–70, https://doi.org/10.1017/S0033291721001975.

22. Jay Joseph, "Inaccuracy and Bias in Textbooks Reporting Psychiatric Research: The Case of the Schizophrenia Adoption Studies," *Politics and the Life Sciences* 19, no. 1 (2000): 89–99, http://www.jstor.org/stable/4236566.

23. American Psychiatric Association, *Resource Document on Neuroimaging* (Washington, DC: American Psychiatric Association, 2018), https://www.psychiatry.org/File%20 Library/Psychiatrists/Directories/Library-and-Archive/resource_documents/2018 -Resource-Neuroimaging.pdf.

24. Emma J. Williams *et al.*, "Telling Lies: The Irrepressible Truth?," *PLoS One* 8, no. 4 (April 2013): e60713, https://doi.org/10.1371/journal.pone.0060713.

25. Hannah Arendt, "Hannah Arendt: From an Interview," *New York Review of Books*, October 26, 1978, https://www.nybooks.com/articles/1978/10/26/hannah-arendt-from-an -interview/.

26. National Institutes of Health, "Information about Mental Illness and the Brain."

27. Cited in Stuart A. Kirk, David Cohen, and Tomi Gomory, "DSM-5: The Delayed Demise of Descriptive Diagnosis," in *The DSM-5 in Perspective. History, Philosophy and Theory of the Life Sciences*, ed. Steeves Demazeux and Patrick Singy (Dordrecht: Springer, 2015), 63–82.

28. Andrew C. Leon *et al.*, "False Positive Results: A Challenge for Psychiatric Screening in Primary Care," *American Journal of Psychiatry* 154, no. 10 (October 1997): 1462–64, https://ajp.psychiatryonline.org/doi/pdf/10.1176/ajp.154.10.1462; Jerome C. Wakefield, "Psychological Justice: DSM-5, False Positive Diagnosis, and Fair Equality of Opportunity," *Public Affairs Quarterly* 29, no. 1 (January 2015): 32–75, https://www.jstor.org /stable/43574514; Mark Zimmerman, "A Review of 20 Years of Research on Overdiagnosis and Underdiagnosis in the Rhode Island Methods to Improve Diagnostic Assessment and Services (MIDAS) Project," *The Canadian Journal of Psychiatry* 61,

no. 2 (February 2016): 71–79, https://doi.org/10.1177/0706743715625935; Eva Charlotte Merten *et al.*, "Overdiagnosis of Mental Disorders in Children and Adolescents (in Developed Countries)," *Child and Adolescent Psychiatry and Mental Health* 11, (January 2017): article 5, https://doi.org/10.1186/s13034-016-0140-5; "Over-Diagnosis and Over-Treatment of Depression Is Common in the U.S.," John Hopkins Bloomberg School of Public Health, April 30, 2013, https://www.jhsph.edu/news/news-releases/2013 /mojtabai-depression-over-diagnosis-and-over-treatment.html; Wakefield, "DSM-5, Psychiatric Epidemiology and the False Positives Problem;" Jerome C. Wakefield, "Diagnostic Issues and Controversies in DSM-5: Return of the False Positives Problem," *Annual Review of Clinical Psychology* 12 (March 2016): 105–32, https://doi .org/10.1146/annurev-clinpsy-032814-112800.

29. Amy Harmon, "A Specialists' Debate on Autism Has Many Worried Observers: National Desk," *New York Times*, January 21, 2012, https://www.nytimes.com/2012/01/21 /us/as-specialists-debate-autism-some-parents-watch-closely.html.

30. R. J. Reinhart, "Nurses Continue to Rate Highest in Honesty, Ethics," *Gallup News Service*, January 6, 2020, https://news.gallup.com/poll/274673/nurses-continue-rate -highest-honesty-ethics.aspx.

31. Open Science Collaboration, "Estimating the Reproducibility of Psychological Science," *Science* 349, no. 6251 (August 2015), https://doi.org/10.1126/science.aac4716; R. Brian Haynes, "Bmjupdates+, a New Free Service for Evidence-Based Clinical Practice," *Evidence-Based Nursing* 8, no. 2 (2005): 39, https://doi.org/10.1136/ebn.8 .2.39; John P. A. Ioannidis, "Why Most Published Research Findings Are False," *PLoS Medicine* 2, no. 8 (August 2005): e124, https://doi.org/10.1371/journal.pmed.0020124; Despina G. Contopoulos-Ioannidis, Evangelia Ntzani, and John P. A. Ioannidis, "Translation of Highly Promising Basic Science Research into Clinical Applications," *American Journal of Medicine* 114, no. 6 (April 2003): 477–84, https://doi.org/10.1016 /s0002-9343(03)00013-5; Yudhijit Bhattacharjee, "The Mind of a Con Man," *The New York Times Magazine*, April 26, 2013, https://www.nytimes.com/2013/04/28/magazine /diederik-stapels-audacious-academic-fraud.html; "How Science Can Go Off the Rails," Vox.com, 2015, accessed August 2020, https://www.thinglink.com/scene/6550 45035355537409; "How Science Goes Wrong," *The Economist*, October 21, 2013, https://www.economist.com/leaders/2013/10/21/how-science-goes-wrong; Fiona Godlee, Catharine R. Gale, and Christopher N. Martyn, "Effect on the Quality of Peer Review of Blinding Reviewers and Asking Them to Sign Their Reports: A Randomized Controlled Trial," *JAMA* 280, no. 3 (1998): 237–40, https://doi.org/10.1001 /jama.280.3.237; Nattanit Gregoris and Simon Shorvon, "What Is the Enduring Value of Research Publications in Clinical Epilepsy? An Assessment of Papers Published in 1981, 1991, and 2001," *Epilepsy and Behavior* 28, no. 3 (September 2013): 522–29, https://doi.org/10.1016/j.yebeh.2013.03.031; Monya Baker, "First Results from Psychology's Largest Reproducibility Test," *Nature* (April 2015), https://doi.org/10.1038 /nature.2015.17433; Demetris Christopoulos, "Should We Treat a Paid Publication as a Real Scientific Publication?," ResearchGate Questions, December 11, 2013, https:// www.researchgate.net/post/Should_we_treat_a_paid_publication_as_a_real_scientific _publication; Colin F. Camerer *et al.*, "Evaluating the Replicability of Social Science Experiments in *Nature* and *Science* between 2010 and 2015," *Nature Human Behaviour* 2 (2018): 637–44, https://doi.org/10.1038/s41562-018-0399-z; Ed Yong, "Nobel Laureate Challenges Psychologists to Clean Up Their Act," *Nature*, (October 2012), https://doi.org/10.1038/nature.2012.11535.

32. Insel, "Transforming Diagnosis."

33. Cosgrove and Krimsky, "A Comparison of *DSM-IV* and *DSM-5*."

34. Brent Dean Robbins, Sarah R. Kamens, and David N. Elkins, "*DSM-5* Reform Efforts by the Society for Humanistic Psychology," *Journal of Humanistic Psychology* 57, no. 6 (November 2017): 602–24, https://doi.org/10.1177/0022167817698617; Div. 32 (Society for Humanistic Psychology), "Open Letter Regarding the Reform and Revision of Diagnostic Systems," APA Divisions, February 24, 2020, https://www.apadivisions.org /division-32/leadership/task-forces/diagnostic-alternatives.

35. Greenberg, *The Book of Woe*, 349.

36. Sandra Steingard, ed., *Critical Psychiatry: Controversies and Clinical Implications* (Cham, Switzerland: Springer, 2019).

37. Peter Tyrer, "A Comparison of DSM and ICD Classifications of Mental Disorder," *Advances in Psychiatric Treatment* 20, no. 4 (July 2014): 280–85, https://doi.org/10.1192 /apt.bp.113.011296; Scott O. Lilienfeld and Michael T. Treadway, "Clashing Diagnostic Approaches: DSM-ICD Versus RDoC," *Annual Review of Clinical Psychology* 12 (2016): 435–63, https://doi.org/10.1146/annurev-clinpsy-021815-093122; "About RDoC," National Institute of Mental Health, https://www.nimh.nih.gov/research /research-funded-by-nimh/rdoc/about-rdoc.shtml.

38. Michael Vlessides, "The Past, Present, and Future of the DSM," Medscape, December 23, 2020, https://www.medscape.com/viewarticle/942694#vp_6.

39. Jeffrey A. Lieberman, *Shrinks: The Untold Story of Psychiatry* (New York: Little, Brown and Company, 2015), 10, Kindle.

40. Robert Whitaker and Lisa Cosgrove, *Psychiatry Under the Influence: Institutional Corruption, Social Injury, and Prescriptions for Reform* (New York: Palgrave Macmillan, 2015).

41. Jeffrey A. Lieberman, "DSM-5: Caught between Mental Illness Stigma and Anti-Psychiatry Prejudice," MIND Guest Blog, *Scientific American*, May 20, 2013, https:// blogs.scientificamerican.com/mind-guest-blog/dsm-5-caught-between-mental-illness -stigma-and-anti-psychiatry-prejudice/.

42. Judy Stone, "Anti-Psychiatry Prejudice? A Response to Dr. Lieberman," Molecules to Medicine (blog), *Scientific American*, May 24, 2013, https://blogs.scientificamerican .com/molecules-to-medicine/anti-psychiatry-prejudice-a-response-to-dr-lieberman/; Whitaker and Cosgrove, *Psychiatry Under the Influence*.

43. Gardiner Harris, "Drug Maker Told Studies Would Aid It, Papers Say," *New York Times*, March 19, 2009, https://www.nytimes.com/2009/03/20/us/20psych.html.

44. Joel Paris, *The Intelligent Clinician's Guide to the DSM-5* (Oxford: Oxford University Press, 2015), 8, ProQuest Ebook Central.

45. Healthy People 2020, "Mental Health," US Office of Disease Prevention and Health Promotion, accessed December 2, 2021, https://www.healthypeople.gov/2020/leading -health-indicators/2020-lhi-topics/Mental-Health/determinants#1.

46. Kawa and Giordano, "A Brief Historicity"; Allen Frances, "It's Not Too Late to Save 'Normal,'" *Los Angeles Times*, March 1, 2010, https://www.latimes.com/archives/la-xpm -2010-mar-01-la-oe-frances1-2010mar01-story.html.

47. Michael Chmielewski et al., "Method Matters: Understanding Diagnostic Reliability in DSM-IV and DSM-5," *Journal of Abnormal Psychology* 124, no. 3 (2015): 764–69, https://doi.org/10.1037/abn0000069; Robert Freedman et al., "The Initial Field Trials of DSM-5: New Blooms and Old Thorns," *American Journal of Psychiatry* 170, no. 1 (2013): 1–5, https://doi.org/10.1176/appi.ajp.2012.12091189.

Index